Melanoma Research: Genetics, Growth Factors, Metastases, and Antigens

Cancer Treatment and Research

WILLIAM MCGUIRE, *series editor*

Catalona WJ,Ratliff, TL (eds): Urologic Oncology. 1984 ISBN 0-89838-628-4.
Santen RJ, Manni A (eds): Diagnosis and Management of Endocrine-related Tumors. 1984. ISBN 0-89838-636-5.
Costanzi JJ (ed): Clinical Management of Malignant Melanoma. 1984. ISBN 0-89838-656-X.
Wolf GT (ed): Head and Neck Oncology. 1984. ISBN 0-89838-657-8.
Alberts DS, Surwit EA (eds): Ovarian Cancer. 1985. ISBN 0-89838-676-4.
Muggia, FM (ed): Experimental and Clinical Progress in Cancer Chemotherapy. 1985. ISBN 0-89838-679-9.
Higby DJ (ed): Issues in Supportive Care of Cancer Patients. 1986. ISBN 0-89838-816-3.
Surwit EA, Alberts DS (eds): Cervix Cancer. 1987. ISBN 0-89838-822-8.
Jacobs C (ed): Cancers of the Head and Neck. 1987. ISBN 0-89838-825-2.
MacDonald JS (ed): Gastrointestinal Oncology. 1987. ISBN 0-89838-829-5.
Ratliff TL, Catalona WJ (eds): Genitourinary Cancer. 1987. ISBN 0-89838-830-9.
Nathanson L (ed): Basic and Clinical Aspects of Malignant Melanoma. 1987. ISBN 0-89838-856-2.
Muggia FM (ed): Concepts, Clinical Developments, and Therapeutic Advances in Cancer Chemotherapy. 1987. ISBN 0-89838-879-5.
Frankel AE (ed): Immunotoxins. 1988. ISBN 0-89838-984-4.
Bennett JM, Foon KA (eds): Immunologic Approaches to the Classification and Management of Lymphomas and Leukemias. 1988. ISBN 0-89838-355-2.
Osborne CK (ed): Endocrine Therapies in Breast and Prostate Cancer. 1988. ISBN 0-89838-365-X.
Lippman ME, Dickson R (eds): Breast Cancer: Cellular and Molecular Biology. 1988. ISBN 0-89838-368-4.
Kamps WA, Humphrey GB, Poppema S (eds): Hodgkin's Disease in Children: Controversies and Current Practice. 1988. ISBN 0-89838-372-2.
Muggia FM (ed): Cancer Chemotherapy: Concepts, Clinical Investigations and Therapeutic Advances. 1988. ISBN 0-89838-381-1.
Nathanson L (ed): Malignant Melanoma: Biology, Diagnosis, and Therapy. 1988. ISBN 0-89838-384-6.
Pinedo HM, Verweij J (eds): Treatment of Soft Tissue Sarcomas. 1989. ISBN 0-89838-391-9.
Hansen HH (ed): Basic and Clinical Concepts of Lung Cancer. 1989. ISBN 0-7923-0153-6.
Lepor H (ed): Basic and Clinical Concepts of Lung Cancer. 1989. ISBN 0-7923-0153-6.
Lepor H, Ratliff TL (eds): Urologic Oncology. 1989. ISBN 0-7923-0161-7.
Benz C, Liu E. (eds): Oncogenes. 1989. ISBN 0-7923-0237-0.
Ozols RF (ed): Drug Resistance in Cancer Therapy. 1989. ISBN 0-7923-0244-3.
Surwit EA, Alberts DS (eds): Endometrial Cancer. 1989. ISBN 0-7923-0286-9.
Champlin R (ed): Bone Marrow Transplantation. 1990. ISBN 0-7923-0612-0.
Goldenberg D (ed): Cancer Imaging with Radiolabeled Antibodies. 1990. ISBN 0-7923-0631-7.
Jacobs C (ed): Carcinomas of the Head and Neck. 1990. ISBN 0-7923-0668-6.
Lippman ME, Dickson R (eds): Cellular and Molecular Biology of Breast Cancer 1990. ISBN 0-7923-0868-9.
Nathanson L (ed): Malignant Melanoma: Genetics, Growth Factors, Metastases, and Antigens. 1991. ISBN 0-7923-0895-6.

Melanoma Research: Genetics, Growth Factors, Metastases, and Antigens

edited by

Larry Nathanson
Winthrop-University Hospital
Mineola, New York

SPRINGER SCIENCE+BUSINESS MEDIA, LLC

Cancer Treatment and Research is indexed in the National Library of Medicine MEDLARS System

Library of Congress Cataloging-in-Publication Data

Melanoma research: genetics, growth factors, metastases, and antigens/
edited by Larry Nathanson.
p. cm.—(Cancer treatment and research : CTAR 54)
Includes bibliographical references.
Includes index.
ISBN 978-0-7923-0895-9 ISBN 978-1-4615-3938-4 (eBook)
DOI 10.1007/978-1-4615-3938-4
1. Melanoma—Genetic aspects. 2. Melanoma—Immunological aspects. 3. Growth factors. 4. Matastasis. 5. Tumor antigens.
I. Nathanson, Larry, 1928– II. Series.
(DNLM: 1. Antigens, Neoplasm. 2. Growth Substances—physiology. 3. Melanoma—genetics. 4. Melanoma—immunology.
5. Neoplasm metastases. WA CA693 v. 54 / QZ 200 M5175)
RC280.M37M45 1991
616.99'477—dc20 90-14151
CIP

Originally published by Kluwer Academic Publishers in 1991

Printed on acid-free paper

For my brother, Neal Nathanson, M.D., who first suggested medicine to me as a profession and whose achievements I have often attempted to emulate.

Contents

Cancer Treatment and Research

Foreword

Where do you begin to look for a recent, authoritative article on the diagnosis or management of a particular malignancy? The few general oncology textbooks are generally out of date. Single papers in specialized journal are informative but seldom comprehensive; these are more often preliminary reports on a very limited number of patients. Certain general journals frequently publish good in-depth reviews of cancer topics, and published symposium lectures are often the best overviews available. Unfortunately, these reviews and supplements appear sporadically, and the reader can never be sure when a topic of special interest will be covered.

Cancer Treatment and Research is a series of authoritative volumes that aim to meet this need. It is an attempt to establish a critical mass of oncology literature covering virtually all oncology topics, revised frequently to keep the coverage up to date, and easily available on a single library shelf or by a single personal subscription.

We have approached the problem in the following fashion: first, by dividing the oncology literature into specific subdivisions such as lung cancer, genitourinary cancer, pediatric oncology, etc.; and second, by asking eminent authorities in each of these areas to edit a volume on the specific topic on an annual or biannual basis. Each topic and tumor type is covered in a volume appearing frequently and predictably, discussing current diagnosis, staging, markers, all forms of treatment modalities, basic biology, and more.

In *Cancer Treatment and Research*, we have an outstanding group of editors, each having made a major commitment to bring to this new series the very best literature in his or her field. Kluwer Academic Publishers has made an equally major commitment to the rapid publication of high-quality books and to worldwide distribution.

Where can you go to find quickly a recent authoritative article on any major oncology problem? We hope that *Cancer Treatment and Research* provides an answer.

WILLIAM L. MCGUIRE
Series Editor

Preface

The past few years have seen a qualitative increase in our understanding of molecular genetics and cytogenetics. Cytogenetics has given us clues about gross translocations, deletions, and amplifications of genetic material. These gross abnormalities, in turn, have led us to develop molecular genetic probes that allow us to identify some of the mechanisms of carcinogenesis, including deletion of sequences in the genome that may normally inhibit uncontrolled growth, as well as amplification of other regions that may code for such growth. Furthermore, whereas previous studies in this area had been primarily devoted to malignancies of the myeloproliferative and lymphoproliferative varieties, these studies are now increasingly directed towards the analysis of solid tumors such as malignant melanoma.

In the first chapter, Cowan and Francke give us insight into cytogenetic abnormalities in melanoma, as well as its associated benign marker lesion, the dysplastic nevus. They have focused attention on chromosomes 1, 6, 7, 10, and 11 in melanoma cells and have, for the first time, identified possible absent 9 in dysplastic nevi.

Halaban, in the second section of this book, goes on to examine the role of a variety of growth factors and receptors in growth control of normal and malignant melanocytes. Kock, Schwarz, Micksche, and Luger review the role that immunoregulatory and growth regulatory cytokines, as well as tumor growth factors, may play in the biology of malignant melanoma. Coppock, Tansey, Scandelis, and Nathanson are interested in how phorbol esters and other agents that raise the level of cyclic AMP may interact in tumor promotion and growth regulation in melanocytes and malignant melanoma cells. Valyi-Nagi and M. Herlyn review information on processes by which melanocytes may interact with their neighboring basal keratinocytes in such a way as to maintain a stable system that is capable of protecting the epidermis and dermis from the deleterious effect of ultraviolet light.

D. Herlyn, Adachi, Koprowski, and M. Herlyn report some of the mechanisms responsible for the metastatic spread of malignant melanoma. They utilize a human malignant cell line in a nude mouse model. The authors examine enzymatics, growth factors, and chromosomal modes, and then demonstrate that monoclonal antibodies to specific ganglioside antigens may inhibit melanoma growth in this system. Schultz looks more carefully at the collagenolytic activity of metalloproteinases and their activity in modulating the metastatic process. Multiple enzymes, including procollagenase and prourikinase, are secreted by tumor cells, and the authors touch on how tissue inhibitor of metallopretinases (TIMP) might effect an inhibition of the process.

Hersey reports in greater detail on the ganglioside antigens (also examined by D. Herlyn et al.) and gives us insight into how the expression of a variety of ganglioside antigens interact with one another and with the expression of such antigens on lymphocytes from lymph nodes harboring metastatic melanoma cells. Murray and Rosenblum further explore the observation that interferons may modulate antigen expression on melanoma cells, as they are known to do in the histocompatibility antigen system. Understanding how interferons and other cytokines may modify antigen expression on the cell surface and antigen shedding may lead to further improvement of our methods of clinical immunotherapy.

This volume emphasizes new developments in the laboratory more than it does clinical studies. I would justify this bias by suggesting that it is a reflection of current melanoma research. Moreover, the clinical advances of the 1990s will come from these emerging research advances. For this reason, I hope that clinicians (among whom I number myself) will find this volume of interest.

Acknowledgments

I would also like to acknowledge the help of Donald L. Coppock, Ph.D. for editorial assistance; Jeffrey K. Smith, Vice President and publisher, and Susan E. Earle, Editorial Assistant, Kluwer Academic; Joan M. McNicholas for secretarial and editorial efforts; all the contributing authors for their promptness in manuscript submission; and, finally, William McGuire for continued encouragement.

Contributing Authors

ADACHI, Koji, Ph.D., The Wistar Institute of Anatomy and Biology, 3601 Spruce Street, Philadelphia, PA 19104

COWAN, Janet M., Ph.D., Department of Radiation and Cellular Oncology, University of Chicago Medical Center, 5841 S. Maryland Avenue, Box 442, Chicago, IL 60637

COPPOCK, Donald L., Ph.D., Oncology Research Laboratory, Winthrop-University Hospital, 222 Station Plaza North, Mineola, NY 11501

FRANCKE, Uta, M.D., Howard Hughes Medical Institute and Departments of Genetics and Pediatrics, Stanford University School of Medicine, Stanford, CA 94305-5428

HALABAN, Ruth, Ph.D., Yale University School of Medicine, Department of Dermatology, 333 Cedar Street, P.O. Box 3333, New Haven, CT 06510

HERLYN, Dorothee, D.V.M., The Wistar Institute of Anatomy and Biology, 3601 Spruce Street, Philadelphia, PA 19104

HERLYN, Meenhard, D.V.M., The Wistar Institute of Anatomy and Biology, 36 Spruce Street, Philadelphia, PA 19104

HERSEY, Peter, FRACP, D.Phil., Oncology & Immunology Unit, 4th Floor, David Maddison Building, Royal Newcastle Hospital, Newcastle, N.S.W. 2300, Australia

KÖCK, Andreas, M.D., Department of Dermatology II, Laboratory of Cell Biology, University of Vienna, Alserstrasses 4, A-1090, Vienna, Austria

KOPROWSKI, Hilary, Ph.D., The Wistar Institute of Anatomy and Biology, 36 Spruce Street, Philadelphia, PA 19014

LUGER, Thomas, M.D., Department of Dermatology II, Laboratory of Cell Biology, University of Vienna, Alserstrasse 4, A-1090, Vienna, Austria

MICKSCHE, M., Ph.D., Department of Dermatology II, Laboratory of Cell Biology, University of Vienna, Alserstrasse 4, A-1090, Vienna, Austria

MURRAY, James L., M.D., University of Texas, M.D. Anderson Cancer Center, 1515 Holcombe Boulevard (Box 041), Houston, TX 77030

NATHANSON, Larry, M.D., Oncology-Hematology Division, Winthrop-University Hospital, 222 Station Plaza North, Suite 300, Mineola, NY 11501

ROSENBLUM, Michael G., Ph.D., University of Texas, M.D. Anderson Cancer Center, 1515 Holcombe Boulevard (Box 041), Houston, TX 77030
SCANDELIS, Susan, R.T., Oncology Research Laboratory, Winthrop-University Hospital, 222 Station Plaza North, Mineola, NY 11501
SCHULTZ, Richard M., Ph.D., Department of Biochemistry, Stritch School of Medicine, Loyola University of Chicago, Maywood, IL 60153
SCHWARZ, T., M.D., Department of Dermatology II, Laboratory of Cell Biology, University of Vienna, Alserstrasse 4, A-1090, Vienna, Austria
TANSEY, Jeanne B., R.T., Oncology Research Laboratory, Winthrop-University Hospital, 222 Station Plaza North, Mineola, NY 11501
VALYI-NAGY, I.T., Ph.D., The Wistar Institute of Anatomy and Biology, 3601 Spruce Street, Philadelphia, PA 19104

I

Genetics of melanoma

1. Cytogenetic analysis in melanoma and nevi

Janet M. Cowan and Uta Francke

1. Introduction

Cytogenetics has proved to be a useful tool in helping to identify regions of the genome in which genes important in malignant transformation may be located. Several research groups have been studying the cytogenetics of melanoma, and other groups have been studying the molecular changes in transformed melanocytes, but no consensus has been reached on the sequence of events that change normal melanocytes into the aberrant cells found in melanomas. This chapter will review some general background literature (covering solid tumor cytogenetics and the models proposed for transformation) and more specific melanocyte literature, cover briefly the growth of melanocytes, present cytogenetic data from dysplastic nevi and melanomas, and suggest a possible sequence of genetic changes that results in malignancy.

1.1. General background

1.1.1. Cytogenetics. Identification of nonrandom chromosome changes in solid tumors requires careful observation of a number of tumors of the same histological type, since the karyotype abnormalities observed tend to be complex. The final karyotype is a mixture of changes that are essential for transformation, changes that add growth advantages but that are not essential, and changes that happen by change and have a neutral effect [1]. For a change to be described as essential for transformation, it must be seen as the sole anomaly in a proportion of cases at an early stage [1]. The changes resulting in growth advantages are often nonrandom and show clonal evolution, while the incidental changes tend to be nonclonal.

In leukemia nonrandom changes often occur as the sole anomaly [1] and have been used to distinguish subtypes of leukemia whose responses to treatment may differ [reviewed by 2]. Few chromosome changes occur in common among the subtypes, except the occurrance of an additional chromosome 8, which is seen in several subtypes during disease progression [2]. In contrast, many of the chromosomal alterations seen in solid tumors

L. Nathanson (ed.), MELANOMA RESEARCH: GENETICS, GROWTH FACTORS, METASTASES, AND ANTIGENS.

have been observed in diverse tumor types, for instance, duplication of chromosome 7 is a common finding in many types of tumor, and iso(6p) has been reported in retinoblastoma, ovarian cancer, and melanoma [3–5].

From the results reported it is apparent that in the majority of leukemias the characteristic change(s) involves reciprocal translocation(s) [6]. Nonrandom translocations have been reported in some solid tumors, including synovial sarcoma, where the translocation involves chromosomes Xp and 18q [7], Ewing's sarcoma, t(11;22)(q24;q12) [8], and lipoma, in which breakpoints in 12q have been identified, 12q13 and 12q14 [9]. In addition, cytogenetic analysis of solid tumors has shown that many are associated with the nonrandom loss of chromosomal material rather than translocation, for example, chromosome 22 in acoustic neuroma [10] and bands p14–p21 of chromosome 3 in small cell lung cancer [11].

1.1.2. Activation and inactivation of genes. As cytogenetic studies progressed, showing the specificity of chromosomal change, molecular analysis was also progressing. It was found that malignancy could be the result of the alteration or activation of a normal cellular gene, such that the gene product was produced continually, or the product was altered or the product was not produced. Examples of these changes are the c-*myc* oncogene, which is overexpressed in Burkitts lymphoma [12,13]; the c-*abl* oncogene in CML, which forms an abnormally sized protein after translocation [14]; and the retinoblastoma gene, which is inactivated in retinoblastoma [15]. Activated oncogenes have been identified in many tumors [16], and chromosomal translocation has been shown to be one method of activation. Tumors characterized by chromosomal deletion, such as retinoblastoma, acoustic neuroma, and small-cell lung cancer, are considered to be the result of inactivation of a tumor suppressor gene, both copies of which must be inactivated for tumor formation.

1.1.3. How many gene changes are required? The evidence from leukemia and retinoblastoma suggested that a single gene change was all that was necessary for malignancy and that each tumor type would be characterized by one nonrandom chromsome change (translocation or deletion). Additional changes would not be essential, but could provide growth advantages for the cell. This model did not seem to fit well with the observations of solid tumors other than retinoblastoma, since there were often conflicting reports about which nonrandom chromosome change was sufficient for transformation (the literature on melanoma is a good example). Many of these questions were answered by a study of colorectal cancer, in which a variety of chromosome changes and oncogene activation had been reported [17–22]. The analysis showed that as lesions progress from benign adenomatous polyps to malignant carcinomas, there is an accumulation of genetic changes, none of which alone is sufficient for transformation [23]. The changes include deletion of the long arms of chromosome 5 and 18, and the short arm of chromosome 17, and activation of the k-*ras* oncogene. These observations suggest a combination of both models of malignant transformation-tumor suppressor deletion and oncogene activation.

2. Melanoma background

2.1. Dysplastic nevus syndrome

Individuals with dysplastic nevus syndrome (DNS) have an increased risk of developing melanoma, as do individuals with giant congenital nevi [24,25]. Histological analysis of sections from superficial spreading melanomas showed areas of cells consistent with a preexisting nevus in 5 of 5 cases [26]. These data suggest that melanomas may preferentially arise in the site of a preexisting nevus [27]. Dysplastic nevi may be considered as premalignant or early-malignant lesions, and as such would be expected to exhibit chromosome changes that are essential for malignant transformation.

It has recently been reported that a gene for hereditary cutaneous malignant melanoma-DNS maps to the distal part of chromosome 1p [28]; however, other groups have been unable to confirm this linkage [29].

2.2. Melanocyte cytogenetics

Analysis of melanocytes derived from nonmalignant nevi and malignant melanomas has not identified one sole chromosome region as being consistently involved, but several chromosomes are reported to be nonrandomly rearranged or deleted, including 1, 6, 7, [5,30], 3 and 9]31–33], and 10 [34, 35]. These observations suggest that melanoma may be more like colon cancer than retinoblastoma, and the final malignancy is the result of accumulation of a number of changes. The most frequently reported change is deletion of 6q, often with duplication of 6p; additional copies of 7, particularly 7p, are also frequently observed in advanced tumors [36]; chromosome 1 is frequently involved in translocation and duplication of the long arm, and it has been suggested that loss of sequences from 1p is a late event in disease progression [37].

Melanoma of the eye is a rare occurrence, but several cases have been studied cytogenetically. Griffin et al. [38] reported a case with the karyotype 46, XY, −21, +t(6p21q), resulting in trisomy of 6p, similar to findings in cutaneous melanoma. However, molecular studies (see below) suggest that uveal melanoma and cutaneous melanoma may have different etiologies.

2.3. Molecular analyses of melanoma

Two groups have reported results of screening melanomas for loss of heterozygosity, one in uveal melanoma [39] and the other in nonuveal melanoma [40]. The first study examined loci on every autosome and only found loss of heterozygosity for loci on chromosome 2p. The second study tested loci on chromosomes 1, 3, 5, 7, 10, 13, 15, 17, 18, 20, and 22, and found the overall rate of loss of heterozygosity was 27% and there was no clear pattern to the losses. Thus the results of molecular analysis mirror those of cytogenetic analysis in showing that melanocyte transformation is a complex process.

3. Culture methods

3.1. *Dysplastic nevi*

Melanocytes derived from dysplastic nevi require other growth factors, in addition to those present in fetal calf serum [41]. One of the most important factors is basic fibroblast growth factor [42], which can be substituted by TPA (12-O-tetradecanoyl-phorbol-13-acetate) in culture. In addition, stimulation of cyclic AMP is also required, and can be achieved with IBMX (isobutyl-methyl xanthine). When grown in this medium, the cells have a characteristic dendritic appearance and will undergo several rounds of replication. Figure 1A shows melanocytes in culture, compared with fibroblasts (Figure 1C).

3.2. *Primary melanoma melanocytes*

The growth requirements of melanocytes from primary melanomas fall between those of melanocytes from dysplastic nevi and metastatic melanomas. Some require TPA and IBMX at the same concentrations, while others will only grow in much lower concentrations (50–90% lower). Cytogenetic analysis of melanocytes from primary melanomas have rarely been reported, due in part to the problems associated with establishing the cells in culture. The morphology of primary melanocytes tends to be bipolar rather than dendritic, with shorter cellular projections and larger nuclei than normal melanocytes (not illustrated).

3.3. *Metastatic melanoma*

Melanocytes from metastatic melanomas are among the easiest cells to establish in culture. The cells will grow well in media supplemented solely with 15–20% fetal calf serum. Figure 1B shows the appearance of these melanocytes in culture. Note the loss of the dendritic form in the majority of cells, and a more fibroblastlike appearance.

3.4. *Pure melanocyte populations*

One problem with analysis of cells derived from solid tumors is contamination of the culture with fibroblasts derived from the stroma of the tumor. From

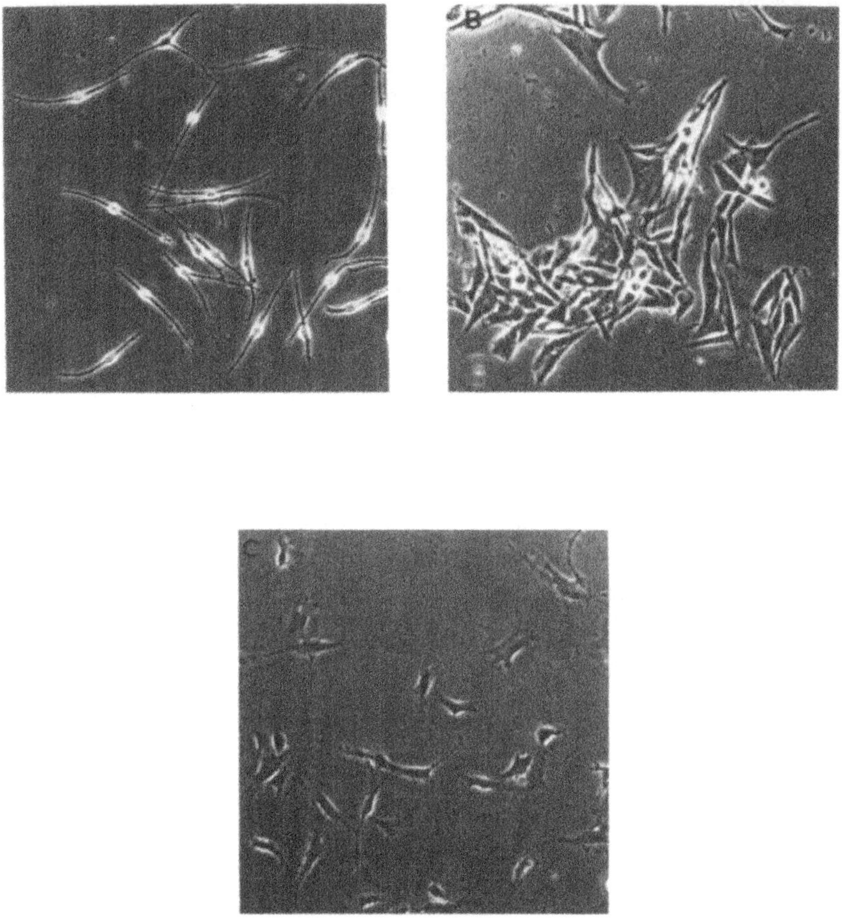

Figure 1. A. Characteristic appearance of normal melanocytes (derived from foreskin) in culture. B. Melanocytes from a mestastatic melanoma in culture. C. Fibroblasts growing in a culture derived from a congenital nevus.

Figure 1 it can be seen that the different cell types can be readily distinguished. Early in the establishment of cultures, fibroblasts can help the melanocytes to grow. However, for cytogenetic analysis a pure population of cells is preferable. For normal melanocytes and melanocytes from primary melanomas, this can be achieved by knocking the flask or by vigorous pipetting. The melanocytes will float off, leaving the fibroblasts behind. Melanocytes from metastatic lesions are more firmly attached (see Figure 1) and will not detach as readily. Treatment of the culture will G418 sulfate (geneticin) for 3 days, followed by washing and reincubation in fresh medium, will result in fibroblast death within 7–10 days [43].

4. Results

Cytogenetic analysis can provide two sets of data. The first is the identification of chromosomal bands that are frequently involved in rearrangement and may pinpoint the site of gene activation. Other useful information includes the frequencies and sites of chromosomal duplication or deletion, which may highlight a region in which a tumor suppressor gene may be located. In order to try to shed new light on the problems associated with the data from melanocyte analysis, we present our results in both ways.

We have previously reported results of the analysis of a large series of

Table 1. Number of samples showing duplication (dup) or deletion (del) for each autosome arm observed in four dysplastic nevi (DN) and 14 melanomas (MEL)

Chrom.	p dup DN	MEL	q dup DN	MEL	p del DN	MEL	q del DN	MEL
1	0	2*	0	**7**	0	1	0	2*
2	0	0	0	0	0	5	0	4
3	0	4*	0	3*	0	1	0	1
4	0	0	0	0	1	2	1	2
5	0	2	0	1	0	1	0	3*
6	0	4	0	2	0	2	0	**8***
7	1	**9**	1	**8**	0	0	0	0
8	1	6	0	**8**	0	1	0	1
9	0	1	0	3	**2**	**9***	**2**	4
10	0	0	0	0	0	**10***	0	**8***
11	1	0	1	0	0	6	0	**9***
12	0	2	0	2*	0	3	0	4*
13	0	0	0	2	0	0	0	2
14	0	0	0	0	0	0	0	6*
15	0	0	0	1	0	0	0	2
16	0	3	0	3	0	3	1	**7**
17	0	1	0	2	0	1	0	1
18	1	1	0	3	0	3	0	2
19	0	3	0	3	0	2	0	1
20	0	**7**	1	**7**	0	1	0	1
21	1	1	1	2	0	1	0	1
22	0	0	0	**7**	0	0	0	1

Frequencies equal to 50% or greater are indicated in bold type. 0 indicates ploidy; * indicates not all of the arm duplicated or deleted.

Chromosome 1	dup: 1 line only cent → p13; del: 1 line only q42 → qter.
Chromosome 3	dup: 1 line only p13 → pter; 1 line only cent → q23, 1 line only q25 → qter.
Chromosome 5	del: 2 lines only q31 → qter.
Chromosome 6	del: all breakpoints between cent and q15.
Chromosome 9	del: 2 lines only p22 → pter.
Chromosome 10	del: 1 line only p15 → pter; del: 1 line only q24 → qter, 1 line interstitial del q22.3 → q24.1.
Chromosome 11	del: 1 line only q23 → qter, 1 line only q21 or q23 → qter; 1 possible interstitial deletion q21 → q23.
Chromosome 12	dup: 1 line cent → q22; del: 1 line q24.1 → qter.
Chromosome 14	del: 1 line q24 → qter, 1 line q13 → qter.

melanocytes from congenital and dysplastic nevi, primary melanoma, and metastatic melanoma [31]. An additional five melanoma samples have been added to the series for this analysis. The three samples from patient 5 of the previous series were treated as one sample, and loss or gain was included if observed in 2 of the 3 samples. While additional dysplastic nevi have been analyzed in the interim, all had normal karyotypes.

Table 1 lists the frequency of loss or duplication of chromosomal material observed in the karyotypes of patients previously reported and of, five additional melanoma samples. The results from the melanoma samples are illustrated in Figure 2. Loss of X and Y chromosomes was not recorded, since one of these chromosomes is often lost in mitoses from cultures of lymphocytes of older individuals, and also in many solid tumor samples (typically an X in females and a Y in males; loss of an X is less common in males). Additionally, when a sample from a male appears to be triploid, the karyotype can be XXY or XYY, and when only one X and Y are present, scoring which has been lost would be guesswork.

From this table it can be seen that several chromosomes are frequently (50% of samples or more) duplicated in the melanomas analyzed: 1q, 7p, 7q, 8q, 20p, 20q, and 22q. Frequent deletion was observed for the following regions: 6q, 9p, 10p, 10q, 11q, and 16q. In the dysplastic nevi, the only

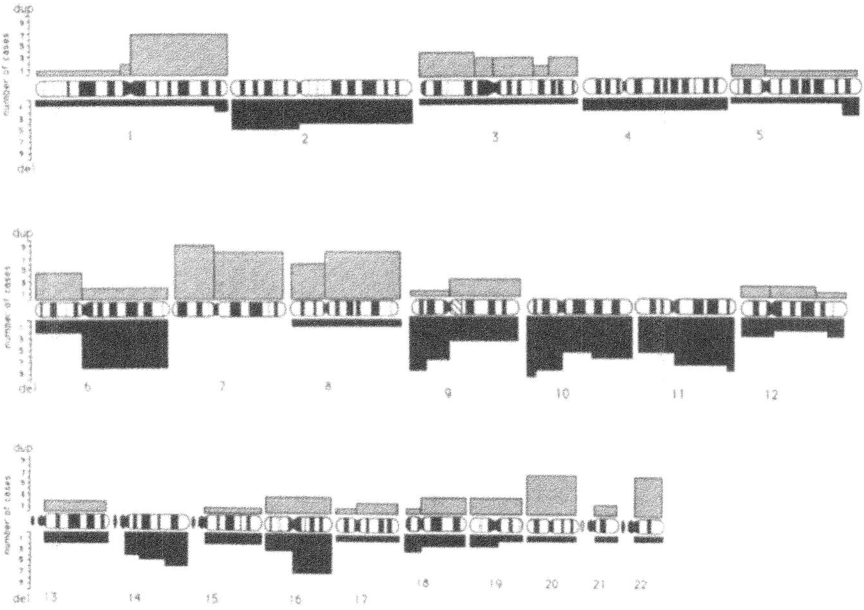

Figure 2. Ideogram showing the frequency of duplication and deletion of chromosomal material in 14 melanomas analyzed. Hatched areas above the chromosome represent duplication; solid areas below the chromosome represent deletion.

significant deletions observed were of 9p and 9q. Chromosome 7 was only duplicated, and chromosomes 2, 4, 10, and 14 were only deleted and not duplicated. Some chromosome regions were duplicated and deleted with nearly equal frequency: 9q, 12p, 13, 15, 16p, 17, 18q, 19p, and 21.

Figure 3 shows the location of all the breakpoints identified in this series of melanocyte samples (nevi and melanoma). It can be seen that several chromosomes have breakpoints clustered in one or two bands. The location of each breakpoint cluster is given in Table 2.

Most of the breaks occurred in heterochromatin regions that contain repetitive DNA, around the centromere, and on the short arms of acrocentrics. Some euchromatic breakpoint clusters occur in regions that are

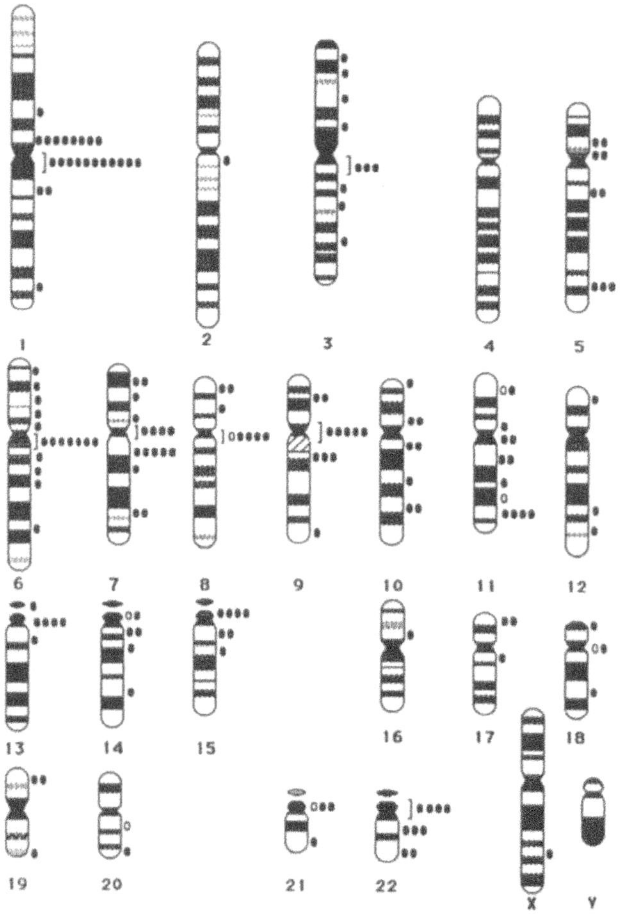

Figure 3. Ideogram showing the location of 163 breakpoints identified in the analysis of four dysplastic nevi and 14 melanomas. Open dots are nevus breakpoints; solid dots are melanoma breakpoints.

Table 2. Distribution of 163 breakpoints observed in melanocyte samples, by chromosome[a]

Chromosome	Total # breaks	Number spfc breaks[b] (%)	Band location
1	22	8 (36)	1p13
2	1	–	–
3	10	–	–
4	0	–	–
5	9	3 (33)	5q33
6	16	6 (37.5)	6q13
7	16	5 (31)	7q11.2
8	8	–	–
9	11	3 (27)	9q13
10	8	–	–
11	13	4 (31)	11q23
12	3	–	–
13	6	4 (67)	13p11.2
14	6	–	–
15	7	4 (57)	15p11.2
16	1	–	–
17	3	2 (67)	17p13
18	4	–	–
19	3	2 (67)	19p13.3
20	2	–	–
21	4	3 (75)	21p11.2
22	9	3 (33)	22q11.2
X	1	–	–

[a]None observed in Y.
[b]Number of specific breakpoints (percentage of total in chromosome).

deleted distal to the breakpoint (5q33, 6q13, 11q23). The breakpoint observed on 7q leads to the duplication of 7q, while that in 9 leads equally to deletion and duplication in the melanoma samples. There appears to be frequent involvement of the short arms of the acrocentric chromosomes, with the exception of chromosome 14.

5. Discussion

The data presented here, from four dysplastic nevi and 14 melanomas, are in general agreement with the data from the literature, with two exceptions. We found few rearrangements involving chromosomes 2 or 3, in contrast to the report by Pedersen et al. [32,33], and the combined number of breakpoints in the two chromosomes was lower than that on several other smaller chromosomes (e.g., 6, 7, 9, 11).

In considering the data for identification of the location of a tumor suppressor gene that must be deleted for transformation, four chromosomes should be considered: 6q, 9p, 10p and q, and 11q. In each case a high proportion of the melanomas showed deletion of these regions. However, the only region showing similar deletion in the dysplastic nevi is 9p. Thus, since dysplastic nevi can be considered precursor lesions for melanoma, we suggest deletion of a gene or genes on 9p to be a primary event in melanocyte transformation, though not necessarily sufficient for malignant progression. Deletion of additional tumor suppressor genes from other shromosomal regions probably occurs in the order 10p, 11q, and then 10q and 6q equally. Since there appears to be a breakpoint hot spot in 11q23, within a region preferentially deleted, alteration of this region may occur before deletion of 10p. Activation of an oncogene in 1p13 is also likely to be a contributing event.

It was recently reported that the addition of a human chromosome 6 to two melanoma cell lines resulted in the loss of their tumor-forming ability in nude mice [44]. Chromosome 6 was added to the cells by microcell fusion, and the resultant hybrids showed different in-vitro growth characteristics from the parental lines, and in addition failed to form tumors when injected into nude mice. Tumor-forming ability returned when one of the hybrid lines lost the fusion chromosome 6. This result is not incompatible with the proposed sequence of events outlined above. If melanocyte malignancy is the result of deletion of a number of tumor suppressor genes, the replacement of any one of those genes may be sufficient for the loss of tumor formation in nude mice. Alternatively, the loss of sequences on chromosome 6 may be the final event that commits the melanocyte to malignancy and metastasis. Further similar experiments using different chromosomes may clarify these observations.

Parmiter et al. [34,35] have previously suggested that 10q24 → q26 is the site of a gene involved in the early stages of melanocyte neoplasia, based on their observation of a dysplastic nevus with t(9;10)(p24;q24), a metastatic melanoma with t(5;6;10), and the loss of one or more copies of chromosome 10 in 18 of 58 cases of melanoma [35]. Since one of their cases involves 9p, it is equally possible that the gene of interest resides in this region. Priest et al. [45] found 4 of 6 breakpoints on chromosome 9 to be in the short arm and less than two normal copies of chromosome 9 in the majority of their samples, which is in agreement with the data presented here. Chromosomes 10 and 11 were less often deleted in their series.

In the molecular screening reported by Dracopoli et al. [40], loss of heterozygosity for D10S1 (which has been mapped to 10q21–23) was found in 5 of 20 cases. There was no loss of heterozygosity in three cases, and the remaining samples were uninformative. This result suggests that deletion of 10q is unlikely to be a primary event in all melanomas, but may be in some. However, microdeletions of smaller regions of 10q, rather than the total loss of the region, cannot be ruled out. A later study by the same group [46] examined six independent metastases from one patient and found loss of heterozygosity at a locus on 9p in all the samples, suggesting that loss of this region occurred as an early event. The only other loci showing loss of heterozygosity in all the samples mapped to the X chromosome, suggesting that one chromosome X had been lost from the tumor. In this case, the loci examined on chromosome 10 were uninformative.

The involvement of the short arms of 4 of 5 pairs of acrocentrics in rearrangement is interesting, since these are the regions to which the major rRNA genes have been mapped [47]. The rRNA genes are present in multiple copies at each location [48], though usually not all clusters are transcriptionally active, as determined by silver nitrate staining [47]. Thus, the loss of two or three sets through translocation is unlikely to disturb the functioning of the cell. It is interesting that Priest el al. [45] observed a similar pattern of involvement of the acrocentric short arms, with comparatively few rearrangements involving 14p.

5. Summary

We have presented data from the cytogenetic analysis of melanocytes derived from four dysplastic nevi and 14 melanomas. We have confirmed previous results from melanomas, including the loss of chromosome 6q and duplication of 1q and 7p. We did not observe an excess of rearrangements involving chromosomes 2 and 3, but we found frequent deletion of chromosomes 9p, 10p, 10q, and 11q. We observed the loss of chromosome 9 in 2 of 4 dysplastic nevi, and combining this observation with that from the melanomas suggests that deletion or inactivation of a gene on 9p may be a primary event in melanocyte transformation. Other tumor suppressor genes are likely to be involved in the transformation process, and these are most likely located on 10p, 10q, 11q, and 6q. We observed many rearrangement involving chromosome band 1p13 and suggest that activation of a gene in that band may also contribute to the transformation process.

Acknowledgments

We would like to thank Tim Wong and Karen L. Mason for technical assistance, Dr. Ruth Halaban for one of the additional melanoma lines, and Dr. Michelle LeBeau for the computer program containing the chromosome ideograms. The work in U.F.'s laboratory was supported by research grant GM 26105. J.M.C. is supported in part by the Passis Fund and U.F. is an investigator of the Howard Hughes Medical Institute.

References

1. Mitelman, F., Heim, S. (1988) Consistent involvement of only 71 of the 329 chromosomal bands of the human genome in primary neoplasia-associated rearrangements. Cancer Res. 45:7115–7119.
2. Pearson, M., Rowley, J.D. (1985) The relation of oncogenesis and cytogenetics in leukemia and lymphoma (review). Annu. Rev. Med. 36:471–483.
3. Squire, J., Phillips, R.A., Boyce S., Godbout, R., Rogers, B., Gallie, B.L. (1984) Isochromosome 6p, a unique chromosomal abnormality in retinoblastoma: Verification by

standard staining techniques, new densitometric method, and somatic hybridization. Hum. Genet. 66:46–53.
4. Atkin, N.B., Baker, M.C. (1987) Abnormal chromosomes including small metacentrics in 14 ovarian cancers. Cancer Genet. Cytogenet. 26:355–361.
5. Cowan, J.M., Halaban, R., Lane, A.T., Francke, U. (1986) The involvement of 6p in melanoma. Cancer Genet. Cytogenet. 20:255–261.
6. 6th International Workshop on Chromosomes in Leukemia, England, May 11–18, 1987. Cancer Genet. Cytogenet. 40:141–147.
7. Turc-Carel, C., Cin, P.D., Limon, J., Rao, U., Li, F.P., Corson, J.M., Zimmerman, R., Parry, D.M., Cowan, J.M., Sandberg, A.A. (1987) Involvement of chromosome X in primary cytogenetic change in human neoplasia: Nonrandom translocation in synovial sarcoma. Proc. Natl. Acad. Sci. USA 84:1981–1985.
8. Turc-Carel, C., Philip, I., Berger, M-P., Philip, T., Lenoir, G.M. (1983) Chromosome study of Ewing's sarcoma (ES) cell lines. Consistency of a reciprocal translocation t(11;22)(q24;q12). Cancer Genet. Cytogenet. 12:1–19.
9. Mandahl, N., Heim, S., Johansson, B., Bennet, K., Mertens, F., Olsson, G., Rooser, B., Rydholm, A., Willen, H., Mitelman, F. (1987) Lipomas have characteristic structural rearrangements of 12q13–q14. Int. J. Cancer 39:685–688.
10. Seizinger, B.R., Martuza, R.L., Gusella, J.F. (1986) Loss of genes on chromosome 22 in tumorigenesis of human acoustic neuroma. Nature (London) 322:644–647.
11. Whang-Peng, J., Kao-Shan, C.S., Lee, E.C., Bunn, P.A., Carney, D.N., Gazdar, A.F., Minna, J.D. (1982) Specific chromosome defect associated with human small-cell lung cancer; deletion 3p(14–23). Science 215:181–182.
12. Croce, C.M., Thierfelder, W., Erikson, J., Nishikura, K., Finan, J., Lenoir, G.M., Nowell, P.C. (1983) Transcriptional activation of an unrearranged and untranslocated c-*myc* oncogene by translocation of a C lambda locus in Burkitt lymphoma cells. Proc. Natl. Acad. Sci. USA 80:6922–6926.
13. Erikson, J., Nishikura, K., Ar-Rushdi, A., Finan, J., Emanuel, B., Lenoir, G., Nowell, P.C., Croce, C.M. (1983) Translocation of an immunoglobulin kappa locus to a region 3' of an unrearranged c-*myc* oncogene enhances c-*myc* expression. Proc. Natl. Acad. Sci. USA 80:7581–7585.
14. Gale, R.P., Canaani, E. (1984) An 8 kilobase RNA transcript in chronic myelogenous leukemia. Proc. Natl. Acad. Sci. USA 81:5648–5652.
15. Cavenee, W.K., Dryja, T.P., Phillips, R.A., Benedict, W.F., Godbout, R., Gallie, B.L., Murphree, A.L., Strong, L.C., and White, R.L. (1983) Expression of recessive alleles by chromosomal mechanisms in retinoblastoma. Nature (London) 305:779–785.
16. Reddy, E.P., Skalka, A.M., Curran, T., eds. (1988) The Oncongene Handbook. Elsevier, Amsterdam.
17. Reichmann, A., Martin, P., Levin, B. (1981) Chromosomal banding patterns in human large bowel cancer. Int. J. Cancer 28:431–440.
18. Solomon, E., Voss, R., Hall, V., Bodmer, W.F., Jass, J.R., Jeffreys, A.J., Lucibello, F.C., Patel, I., Rider, S.H. (1987) Chromosome 5 allele loss in human colorectal carcinomas. Nature 328:616–619.
19. Muleris, M., Salmon, R.J., Zafrani, B., Girodet, J., Dutrillaux, B. (1985) Consistent deficiencies of chromosome 18 and of the short arm of chromosome 17 in eleven cases of human large bowel cancer: A possible recessive determinism. Ann Genet (Paris) 28:206–213.
20. Fearon, E.R., Hamilton, S.R., Vogelstein, B. (1987) Clonal analysis of human colorectal tumors. Science 238:193–197.
21. Bos, J.L., Fearon, E.R., Hamilton, S.R., Verlaan de Vries, M., van Boom, J.H., van der Eb, A.J., Vogelstein, B. (1987) Prevalence of *ras* gene mutations in human colorectal cancers. Nature 327:293–297.
22. Forrester, K., Almoguera, C., Han, K., Grizzle, W.E., Perucho, M. (1987) Detection of K-*ras* oncogenes during human colon tumorigenesis. Nature 327:298–303.

23. Vogelstein, B., Fearon, E.R., Hamilton, S.R., Kern, S.E., Preisinger, A.C., Leppert, M., Nakamura, Y., White, R., Smits, A.M.M., Bos, J.L. (1988) Genetic alterations during colorectal-tumor development. N. Engl. J. Med. 319:525–532.
24. Greene, M.H., Clark, W.H. Jr., Tucker, M.A., Kraemer, K.H., Elder, D.E., Fraser, M.C. (1985) High risk of malignant melanoma in melanoma-prone families with dysplastic nevi. Ann. Intern. Med. 102:458–465.
25. Hendrickson, M.R., Ross, J.C. (1981) Neoplasms arising in giant congenital nevi. Am. J. Surg. Pathol. 5:109–135.
26. Elder, D.E., Goldman, L.I., Goldman, S.C., Greene, M.H., Clark, W.H. (1980) Dysplastic nevus syndrome: A phenotypic association of sporadic cutaneous melanoma. Cancer 46:1787–1794.
27. Green, A., MacLennan, R., Siskind, V. (1985) Common acquired nevi and the risk of malignant melanoma. Int. J. Cancer 35:297–300.
28. Bale, S.J., Dracopoli, N.C., Tucker, M.A., Clark, W.H., Fraser, M.C., Stanger, B.Z., Green, P., Donis-Keller, H., Housman, D.E., Greene, M.H. (1989) Mapping the gene for hereditary cutaneous malignant melanoma-dysplastic nevus to chromosome 1. N. Engl. J. Med. 320:1367–1372.
29. van Haeringen, A., Bergman, W., Nelen, M.R., van der Kooij-Meijs, E., Hendrikse, I., Wijnen, J.T., Meera Khan, P., Klasen, E.C., Frants, R.R. (1989) Exclusion of the dysplastic nevus syndrome (DNS) locus from the short arm of chromosome 1 by linkage studies in Dutch families. Genomics 5:61–64.
30. Limon, J., Dal Cin, P., Sait, S.N., Karakousis, C., Sandberg, A.A. (1988) Chromosome changes in metastatic human melanoma. Cancer Genet. Cytogenet. 30:201–211.
31. Cowan, J.M., Halaban, R., Francke, U. (1988) Cytogenetic analysis of melanocytes from premalignant nevi and melanomas. J. Natl. Cancer Inst. 80:1159–1164.
32. Pedersen, M.I., Bennet, J.W., Wang, N. (1986) Nonrandom chromosome structural aberrations and oncogene loci in human malignant melanoma. Cancer Genet. Ctyogenet. 20:11–27.
33. Pedersen, M.I., Wang, N. (1989) Chromosomal evolution in the progression and metastasis of human malignant melanoma. A multiple lesion study. Cancer Genet. Cytogenet. 41:185–201.
34. Parmiter, A.H., Balaban, G., Clark, W.H., Nowell, P.C. (1988) Possible involvement of the chromosome region 10q24 → q26 in early stages of melanocytic neoplasia. Cancer Genet. Cytogenet. 30:313–317.
35. Parmiter, A.H., Nowell, P.C. (1988) The cytogenetics of human malignant melanoma and premalignant lesions. In: Nathanson L., ed., Malignant Melanoma: Biology, Diagnosis and Therapy. Kluwer Academic, Norwell, MA, pp. 47–61.
36. Koprowski, H., Herlyn, M., Balaban, G., Parmiter, A., Ross, A., Nowell, P. (1985) Expression of the receptor for the epidermal growth factor correlates with increased dosage of chromosome 7 in malignant melanoma. Somat. Cell Mol. Genet. 11:297–302.
37. Dracopoli, N.C., Harnett, P., Bale, S.J., Stanger, B.Z., Tucker, M.A., Housman, D.E., Kefford, R.F. (1989) Loss of alleles from the distal short arm of chromosome 1 occurs late in melanoma tumor progression. Proc. Natl. Acad. Sci. USA 86:4614–4618.
38. Griffin, C.A., Long, P.P., Schachat, A.P. (1988) Trisomy 6p in an ocular melanoma. Cancer Genet. Cytogenet. 32:129–132.
39. Mukai, S., Dryja, T.P. (1986) Loss of alleles at polymorphic loci on chromosome 2 in uveal melanoma. Cancer Genet. Cytogenet. 22:45–53.
40. Dracopoli, N.C., Houghton, A.N., Old, L.J. (1985) Loss of polymorphic restriction fragments in malignant melanoma: Implications for tumor heterogeneity. Proc. Natl. Acad. Sci. USA 82:1470–1474.
41. Eisinger, M., Marko, O. (1982) Selective proliferation of normal human melanocytes in vitro in the presence of phorbol ester and cholera toxin. Proc. Natl. Acad. Sci. USA 79:2018–2022.
42. Halaban, R., Ghosh, S., Baird, A. (1987) bFGF is the putative natural growth factor for

human melanocytes. In Vitro Cell Dev. Biol. 23:47–52.

43. Halaban, R., Alfano, F.D. (1984) Selective elimination of fibroblasts from cultures of human melanocytes. In Vitro 20:447–450.
44. Trent, J.M., Stanbridge, E.J., McBride, H.L., Meese, E.U., Casey, G., Araujo, D.E., Witkowski, C.M., Nagle, R.B. (1990) Tumorigenicity in human melanoma cell lines controlled by introduction of human chromosome 6. Science 247:568–571.
45. Priest, J.H., Phillips, C.N., Wang, Y., Richmond, A. (1988) Chromosome and growth factor abnormalities in melanoma. Cancer Genet. Cytogenet. 35:253–262.
46. Dracopoli, N.C., Alhadeff, B., Houghton, A.N., Old, L.J. (1987) Loss of heterozygosity at autosomal and X-linked loci during tumor progression in a patient with melanoma. Cancer Res. 47:3995–4000.
47. Henderson, A.S., Warburton, D., Atwood, K.C. (1972) Location of ribosomal DNA in the human chromosome complement. Proc. Natl. Acad. Sci. USA 69:3394–3398.
48. Wellauer, P.K., Dawid, I.B. (1973) Secondary structure maps of RNA: Processing of HeLa ribosomal RNA. Proc. Natl. Acad. Sci. USA 70:2827–2831.

II

Growth Regulation/Oncogenes

2. Growth factors regulating normal and malignant melanocytes

Ruth Halaban

1. Introduction

Growth factors and growth factor receptors play a critical role in normal growth and development, and their aberrant expression and/or activity has been implicated in neoplastic transformation. A common characteristic of transformed cells is an acquired independence from environmental growth factors that are needed for the proliferation of the nontransformed cell. Such autonomy can be achieved at the level of the growth factor itself, the growth factor receptor, or molecules involved in the transduction of the mitogenic signal from the cell membrane to the nucleus. For example, aberrant, unregulated production of transforming growth factors (TGF-α and TGF-β) [1–3], platelet-derived growth fator (PDGF) [4,5], interleukins (IL-1, IL-2, and IL-3) [6–10], and epidermal growth factor (EGF) [11] with an induction of an autocrine loop was implicated in the maintenance of the transformed state of the respective target cells. Overexpression of the macrophage-colony stimulating factor (M-CSF) receptor, the EGF receptor, receptors homologous to the EGF receptor, or mutations that confer constitutive activity on the receptors have been shown to be oncogenic [12–17]. Several known retroviral oncogenes, such as v-*erb*-B, v-*erb*-A, *fms*, and *neu*, are transduced cellular genes encoding, respectively, the receptors for EGF, thyroid hormone (T_3), macrophage colony stimulating factor (M-CSF), and an as-yet unidentified ligand [18–26]. Therefore, knowledge of the growth factor dependency of the normal cell may be a first step in the identification of a gene or genes expressed aberrantly in the malignant counterpart. Following is an up-to-date summary of the growth factors that are mitogenic for normal human melanocytes and their expression in melanoma cells.

2. Basic FGF and normal human melanocytes

Comparisons of the growth of normal and malignant melanocytes in culture show that melanoma cells continue to proliferate under conditions in which normal melanocytes remain quiescent or die [27]. Melanoma cells from

L. Nathanson (ed.), MELANOMA RESEARCH: GENETICS, GROWTH FACTORS, METASTASES, AND ANTIGENS.

metastatic lesions grow in chemically defined medium in the presence of common growth factors or in routine, serum-supplemented medium. These media also support the growth of nontransformed cells other than melanocytes, such as skin fibroblasts. Normal melanocytes require specific ingredients in addition to common factors present in serum. For a while the only agent known to support melanocyte proliferation was 12-O-tetradecanoyl-phorbol-13-acetate (TPA), supplied in conjunction with substances that increase intracellular levels of cyclic adenosine monophosphate (cAMP), such as cholera toxin, isobutylmethyl xanthine (IBMX), and dibutyryl cAMP (dbcAMP) [28–30].

A critical step in the search for regulatory factors that are biologically significant to melanocytes was the identification of basic fibroblast growth

Table 1. The melanocyte mitogen in melanoma-conditioned media is bFGF

Additions	^{3}H-thymidine incorporation (cpm/well/3 hr)
hrbFGF	19,600
dbcAMP	1,450
dbcAMP + hrbFGF	38,000
Melanoma-conditioned media plus dbcAMP	
Experiment 1	
YU SIT1	1,000
YU SAC2	2,000
YU DAN3	20,000
YU WIL4	2,000
YU MOL5	2,800
YU ZAZ6	500
SK-MEL23	3,800
SK-MEL37	500
SW-614	15,600
WM9	6,000
Experiment 2	
YU DAN3	1,200
YU DAN3 + dbcAMP	13,000
YU DAN3 + dbcAMP + anti-bFGF-(1-24)-ab	1,600
SW614	2,340
SW614 + dbcAMP	23,000
SW614 + anti-bFGF-(1–24)-ab	2,400

Human melanocytes derived from newborn foreskins were seeded in the chemically defined PC-1 medium in 24-well cluster plates (approximately 30,000 cells/well). Additions were 1 ng/ml hrbFGF (human recombinant basic fibroblast growth factor, Chiron), 1.0 mM dbcAMP (dibutyryl adenosine cyclic monophosphate), and 3 day PC-1 conditioned media from melanomas diluted 1:1 with fresh PC-1 medium. Neutralizing antibodies to bFGF [anti-bFGF-(1–24)-ab], 1:100 dilution, were added directly to experimental media. ^{3}H-thymidine incorporation was performed during the last 3 hours of the 24-hour incubation period. Data are the mean of duplicate wells. Notice that the melanocyte mitogen in melanoma-conditioned media is completely neutralized by anti-bFGF antibodies. Antibodies to plasminogen like growth factor did not neutralize the mitogenic activity of melanoma conditioned media (data not shown).

factor (bFGF) as a natural mitogen for melanocytes [31]. In a short-term 24-hour proliferation assay, bFGF alone is sufficient to stimulate normal human melanocytes [reference 27] (Table 1). This mitogenic action is dependent on the quality of bFGF, because in general cAMP stimulators are needed for maximal mitogenicity [27,31]. In long-term proliferation assays, cAMP is always needed to elicit the mitogenic response of melanocytes to bFGF [31 and our unpublished results]. In situ, bFGF appears to be provided to normal melanocytes by the immediate neighboring cells, because normal melanocytes, unlike other cell types that respond to bFGF, do not produce bFGF on their own [32]. The absence of bFGF in normal melanocytes is seen on both the mRNA and protein levels. Melanocytes do not produce the bFGF gene transcript, nor a protein reactive with anti-bFGF-antibodies (Figure 1), or any other mitogen that stimulates their own proliferation [32]. In contrast,

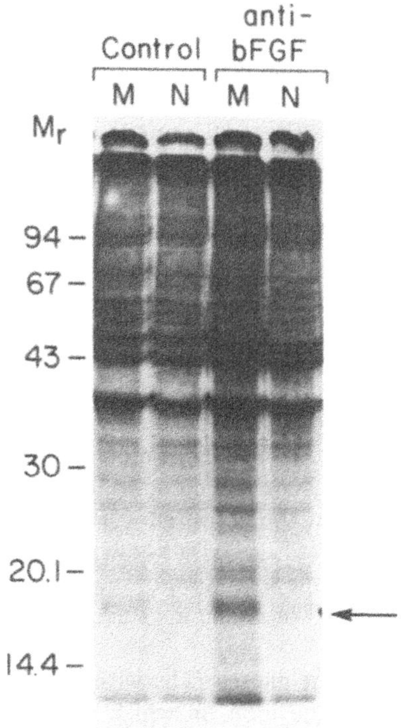

Figure 1. Immunoprecipitated bFGF in melanoma cells. Normal human melanocytes from newborn foreskins (N) and YU SIT1 metastatic melanoma cells (M) were metabolically radiolabeled with ^{35}S-methionine for 6 hours. Extracts containing 5 × 10^7 cpm in TCA perceptible material were subjected to immunoprecipitation by anti-bFGF-(1-24) (anti-bFGF) or by nonimmune rabbit (control) antibodies. Immune complexes were resolved in 15% polyacylamide gels (SDS-PAGE), and gels were fluorographed overnight at room temperature. Molecular size markers ($\times 10^3$) from top to bottom: phosphorylase b, albumin, ovalbumin, carbonic anhydrase, soybean trypsin inhibitor, and lysozyme. Arrow points to bFGF.

other skin cells, such as proliferating keratinocytes and dermal fibroblasts, produce bFGF and in coculture with melanocytes maintain melanocyte viability [33].

3. Expression of bFGF in melanoma cells

The majority of metastatic melanomas and some primary melanomas, particularly those in the vertical growth phase, are independent of melanocyte growth factors because of self-stimulation through aberrant production of bFGF [32]. Metastatic melanoma cells in culture produce mRNA species that hybridize with bFGF cDNA and are similar in size to bFGF mRNA in other cell types [32]. In addition, melanoma cells, but not normal melanocytes, express a protein of about 18 kD, precipitated by anti-bFGF-antibodies (Figure 1). This protein is biologically active because addition of anti-bFGF-antibody neutralizes the mitogenic activity of extracts from cultured melanoma cells toward normal human melanocytes [31,32]. Melanomas are known to express a heparin-binding factor that behaves like bFGF [34–36], and the partially purified melanocyte mitogen in one melanoma cell line was shown to bind heparin [37].

There is evidence that the melanoma cells depend upon this intrinsic mitogen because internalized neutralizing anti-bFGF-antibodies inhibit growth [32]. In addition, antisense, but not sense, oligodeoxynucleotides targeted against three different sites of human bFGF mRNA inhibit proliferation and colony formation in soft agar of metastatic melanoma cells and primary melanoma cells from the vertical growth phase [38]. Antisense oligodeoxynucleotides to nerve growth factor (β-NGF) and insulinlike growth factor I (IGF-I) mRNA had no effect on melanoma cells [38]. An indirect evidence for the importance of bFGF in melanomas growth is the finding that the proliferation of a human melanoma cell line was inhibited by a monoclonal antibody against the active site of urokinase-type plasminogen activator (u-PA) [39]. Because bFGF is known to increase the synthesis of plasminogen activator [40], the inhibition of melanoma growth by anti-u-PA antibody suggests that bFGF in melanomas acts via induction of this serine protease.

The self-stimulation of melanoma cells with bFGF cannot be explained solely by a classical autocrine loop, in which a factor is secreted into the medium and in turn binds to cell surface receptors. Significant levels of bFGF were secreted in only 3 out of 10 melanomas tested (Table 1); in the other cases, the bFGF was cell associated [32,34]. In contrast to classical autocrine loops [41], the self-stimulation of melanoma cells with bFGF cannot be inhibited by the addition of bFGF neutralizing antibodies to the culture medium [32]. Basic FGF lacks a hydrophobic signal peptide that would facilitate its secretion [42,43], yet the peptide must be released, even from normal cells, because it is found in vivo in the extracellular matrix (ECM)

[44,45]. Therefore, it is possible that most of the bFGF produced by melanoma cells in culture is likewise immobilized to the ECM and may not be accessible to neutralizing antibodies in the medium. However, other experiments, discussed below, suggest that bFGF acts in melanomas through an intracellular loop of autocrine stimulation. Precedence for this mechanism exists in the case of *v-sis* (an oncogene derived by transduction of the PDGF-B gene by simian sarcoma virus) [41,46–48], granulocyte/macrophage colony-stimulating factor (GM-CSF), and IL-3 [41,49–51]. The activity of this internal loop in melanoma cells, involving the binding of growth factor to internal bFGF receptors, results in suppression of melanocytic differentiated functions [52]. This internal mode of action is qualitatively different from that of an external autocrine loop, in which the growth factor binds to cell surface receptors and differentiated functions are maintained or even enhanced.

The mechanism by which the bFGF gene becomes expressed in melanomas is not clear. Basic FGF has been mapped to human chromosome 4 [53], which is known to not be affected in melanomas [54–56]. Southern blot analysis suggested that in melanomas the gene is neither amplified nor rearranged [57 and our unpublished results]. However, one should keep in mind that expression of bFGF is a normal event in several tissues in vivo, and in a number of nontransformed cell types in vitro [58], and the expression in melanoma cells, although aberrant for this cell type, is at least 20-fold lower than in normal keratinocytes and skin fibroblasts grown in culture [32,33]. Therefore, suppression of bFGF expression in melanocytes might be an important event leading to their differentiation.

4. Basic FGF receptors

Basic FGF receptor activity in melanomas is critical for proliferation, because synthetic bFGF peptides that span the receptor binding domain and act as bFGF antagonists inhibit melanoma cell growth, whereas peptides from nonrelevant domains have no effect [32]. Internalized anti-phosphotyrosine antibodies also inhibit melanoma cell growth [32]. Both bFGF and aFGF receptors have been shown to be tyrosine kinases [59,60]. The presence of a tyrosine-kinase domain was recently confirmed by cloning of the bFGF and aFGF receptors [61,62,108–111]. The deduced amino acid sequences showed an identity of 51–53% between the two FGF receptor kinase regions and the known tyrosine kinase regions in receptors for PDGF and CSF-1 [61,62, 108–111]. Therefore, the internalized anti-phosphotyrosine antibodies, like the antagonistic peptides, probably inhibit the growth of the cells through inhibition of bFGF receptor activity. The mechanism by which the signal from an activated tyrosine-protein kinase is transmitted to the nucleus is not yet clear. However, it is possible that the activated receptors migrate to the nucleus, because the deduced amino acid sequence of the cloned avian bFGF contains a series of eight consecutive acidic residues that are characteristic of nuclear proteins, suggesting that the human bFGF receptor may have similar properties [61]. In accordance with this hypothesis is the localization of bFGF to nuclear sites [112]. The combined data suggest that the receptor-ligand complex may migrate to the nucleus and exert its mitogenic stimulus in a manner similar to that of transactivating factors.

5. Basic FGF in melanocytes of early melanocytic lesions in vivo and in vitro.

A study on the expression of bFGF in normal skin and melanocytic lesions was recently performed by Scott, Stoler, Sarkar, and Halaban [113]. In-situ hybridization of a riboprobe for bFGF cDNA to sections of normal skin showed the presence of bFGF mRNA in basal keratinocytes (Figure 2). The method did not allow us to determine whether normal melanocytes in vivo produced bFGF. The data on keratinocytes are in accordance with a preceding study showing bFGF gene transcripts only in proliferating and not in stratifying keratinocytes in culture [33]. In the junctional nests of nevic cells, bFGF mRNA was detected at low levels in benign nevi, with an increase in expression in dysplastic nevi, while low expression was observed in the dermal nevic populations of both types of nevi. Medium to high levels of signal were observed in melanocytes of primary melanomas (Figure 2). If benign and dysplastic nevi represent lesions with increased potential toward malignancy, as suggested by Clark and collaborators [63], then one of the initial events in progression towards an autonomous mode of growth could be the aberrant expression of bFGF. However, expression of bFGF by itself is insufficient to confer the malignant phenotype, because melanocytes in common nevi are not malignant. In fact, in patients with the dysplastic nevus syndrome who may have as many as 300 nevi, a single cell in only one dysplastic nevus may give rise to a melanoma. The benign nature of nevus cells expressing bFGF in vivo is in agreement with results obtained by introducing a bFGF cDNA clone into normal melanocytes experimentally [52, and section 6 below].

The low level of expression of bFGF in vivo in nevic melanocytes nevertheless affects the behavior of these cells in culture. Although melanocytes cultured from common and dysplastic nevi generally display complete dependence on melanocyte growth factors, melanocytes derived from two dysplastic nevi from a 28-year-old patient, who had a history of cutaneous melanoma and had the dysplastic nevus syndrome, were able to proliferate in the presence of only cAMP stimulators (in the absence of TPA or bFGF), [27]. In addition, the adult melanocytes from nevi have a longer lifespan in culture than do normal melanocytes and, once growth factors are removed from the medium, they remain viable for a longer period [27]. These data suggest that the low levels of expression of bFGF in nevic melanocytes confer a growth advantage and increased viability under conditions of deprivation that kill normal melanocytes.

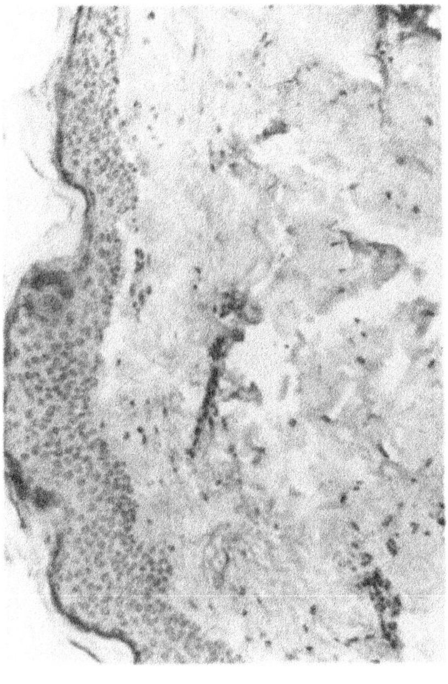

Figure 2A.

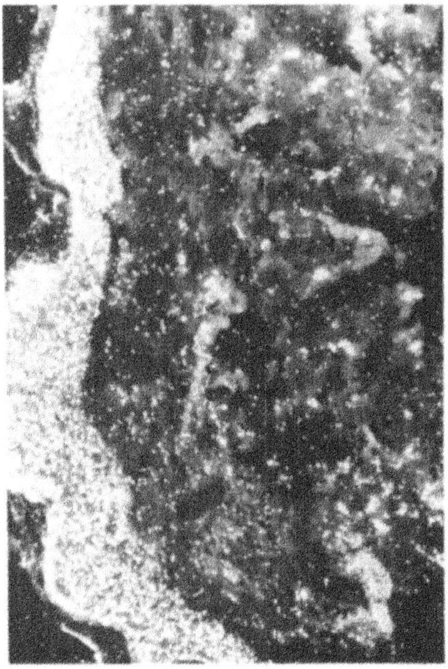

Figure 2A.

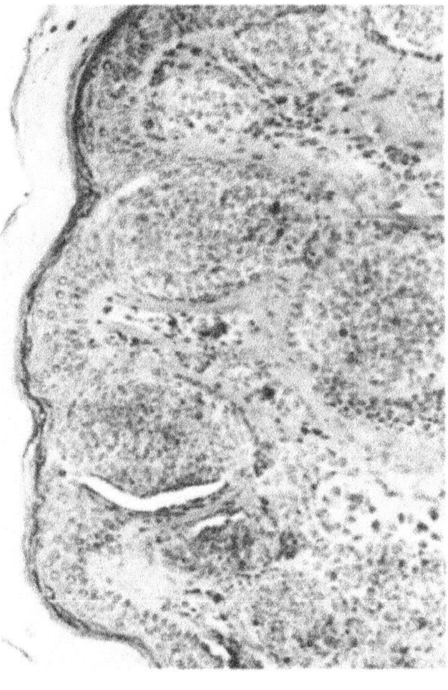

Figure 2B.

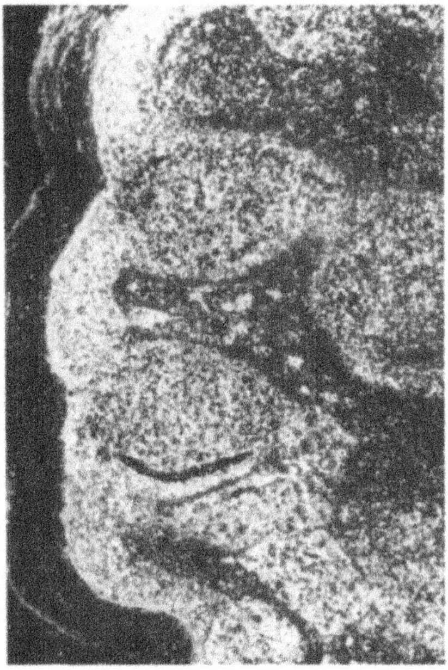

Figure 2B.

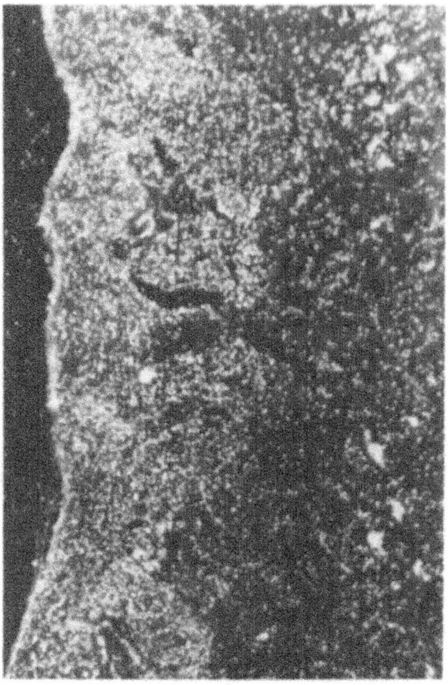

Figure 2C.

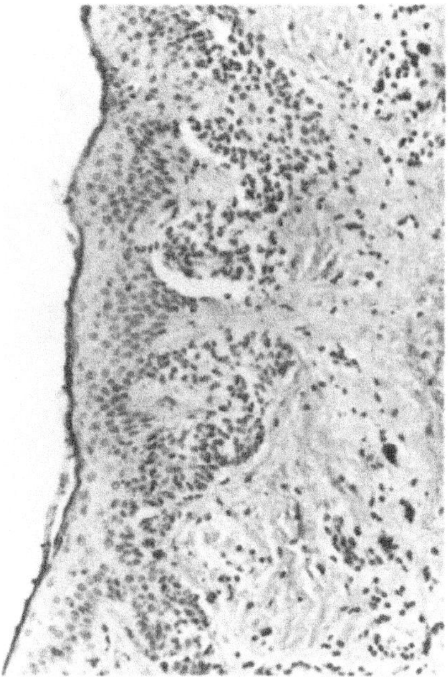

Figure 2C.

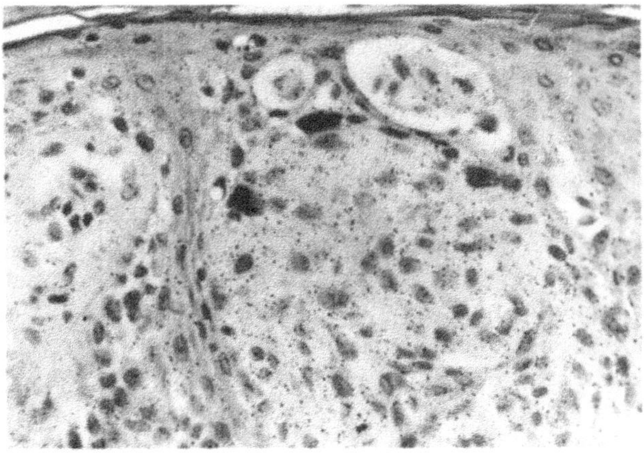

Figure 2D.

Figure 2. Basic FGF mRNA in situ. Excisional biopsies were fixed in 10% formaldehyde, pH 7.4, embedded in paraffin, and sectioned at 4–6 μm. Sections were stained with hematoxylin and eosin. Wax was partially removed by heating to 62°C for 45 minutes before hybridization. Hybridization was performed with a riboprobe prepared from the 1.4-kb bovine cDNA for bFGF [42]. The cDNA was cloned into the *Eco*R1 site of the RNA transcription vector pGEM 3Z. Tritium-labeled asymmetric RNA transcripts were synthesized to a specific activity of 3.7×10^7 cpm/μg. The 'sense' orientation probe was used as a negative control. Hybridization was performed under moderate stringency, washed under high stringency, and followed by autoradiography for 21 days. Left column: Bright field micrograhps. Right column: Dark field micrographs.
A. Normal skin. Normal keratinocytes and fibroblasts show strong hybridization signal (200x). B. Benign compound nevus. Epidermal keratinocytes and junctional nevic cell show strong hybridization signal (200x). C. Dysplastic nevus. Junctional nevic cell show strong hybridization signal (200x). D. Primary malignant melanoma. Malignant melanocytes in the epidermis show hybridization signal (400x).

6. Transformation of a murine melanocyte line with bFGF cDNA and known oncogenes

Experimental manipulation of normal melanocytes to express bFGF constitutively produced results that are in agreement with those described above with in-situ hybridization. The introduction of bFGF cDNA into the murine melanocyte line L-B10.BR via recombinant retroviruses conferred, as expected, autonomous growth in culture [52]. What was not expected was the associated loss of all differentiated functions, including pigmentation, expression of tyrosinase (the key enzyme in melanin synthesis), the synthesis of melanosomes, the subcellular organelles in which melanin is normally deposited, and loss of dendrite formation. The bFGF-transformed melanocytes no longer resembled their original counterpart, but rather appeared like fibroblasts or endothelial cells [52]. In contrast, prolonged exposure of normal melanocytes in culture to bFGF or other mitogens, such as TPA and cAMP stimulators, maintains the cells in a highly differentiated state. In fact, all substances known to stimulate the proliferation of normal melanocytes in culture also stimulate the production of melanocyte-specific mRNAs, tyrosinase, and melanin [64–67]. These observations suggest that differentiation of melanocytes is dependent on continuous cell surface stimulation. Therefore, bFGF produced by the transfected melanocytes probably activates in large part an internal pool of receptors, which effectively maintains the pathway to proliferation, but not to differentiation. It is not clear in which intracellular compartment the endogenous bFGF binds to its receptor since the receptor is a membrane-bound protein, with its receptor domain presumed to be extracytosolic and bFGF is not [42,43,61,62].

The bFGF-transformed melanocytes did not grow as tumors in syngeneic or nude mice. Instead, they regained their differentiated functions, including the ability to produce melanin, and appeared in all respects like normal melanocytes. Thus, expression of bFGF was sufficient to confer autonomous growth in culture, accompanied by extinction of differentiated functions, but did not render the cells tumorigenic. Like the human nevic melanocytes, in vivo, the growth of the bFGF-expressing murine melanocytes was restrained by environmental factors whose nature is not yet known.

When L-B10.BR cells were transformed with *ras* or *neu*, the cells grew as tumors in immunocompetent syngeneic and nude mice, whereas *E1a* and *myc* transformed melanocytes formed tumors only in nude mice [52]. Like the bFGF transformants in vitro, these cells became independent of growth factors and displayed a nonmelanocytic phenotype. Transformation by these oncogenes was not due to activation of bFGF expression, because a melanocyte mitogen could not be detected in these cells. Inhibition of growth by factors produced by adjacent cells in a reconstituted skin environment was evident only in the case of the *neu*-transformants. Tumorigenicity was suppressed when the *neu*-transformants were cografted with keratinocytes. Fibroblasts did not have this effect. Thus, the in-vitro transformed melanocytes demonstrated that tumorigenicity was not solely determined by oncogenes, but also by the immune response and by growth inhibitors produced by neighboring cells.

L-B10.BR melanocytes were not transformed by constitutive expression of mutated p53 [52]. The absence of p53 transforming ability was not due to a defect in the recombinant retroviral vector, because the same construct was able to transform a keratinocyte line [68]. Mutated p53 was recently shown to be suppressed by wild-type p53, suggesting that the latter is a tumor suppressor rather than a tumor promoter [69]. Because in our experiment [52] the p53-transduced melanocytes became neomycin resistant and expressed p53 at higher levels than the original cell line, the absence of transformation may indicate that melanocytes express wild-type p53 and that this gene product counteracted the tumor-promoting effect of the mutated p53.

The originally homogeneous population of murine melanocytes became highly variable in morphology and tumor-forming ability after transformation with oncogenes in vitro. Metastatic melanomas are known to be highly variable with respect to morphology in culture, and expression of cell surface antigens and differentiated functions [70]. Therefore, it is possible that the divergent phenotypes observed in melanomas are due to a diversity in the genetic events operating in each tumor, in addition to the aberrant expression of bFGF. Evidence for heterozygosity of DNA at several loci was recently shown for 24 human melanoma cell lines [55].

7. Transformation of murine melanocytes in primary culture

The results described above were obtained with an immortalized melanocyte line that had already lost the dependency on one growth facor, cAMP. This cell line has an extra chromosome 6 [71]. When similar experiments were performed with primary melanocytes at an early passage (P-B10.BR, passage 6), the outcome was different. These cells incorporated and expressed the recombinant retroviral genes because they became resistant to geneticin due to the expression of the viral neomycin gene. However, the infected cells did not become independent of growth factors and did not loose their melanocytic phenotype [Dotto, Ghosh, and Halaban, unpublished results]. Even the highly transforming *ras* oncogene did not confer autonomous growth to

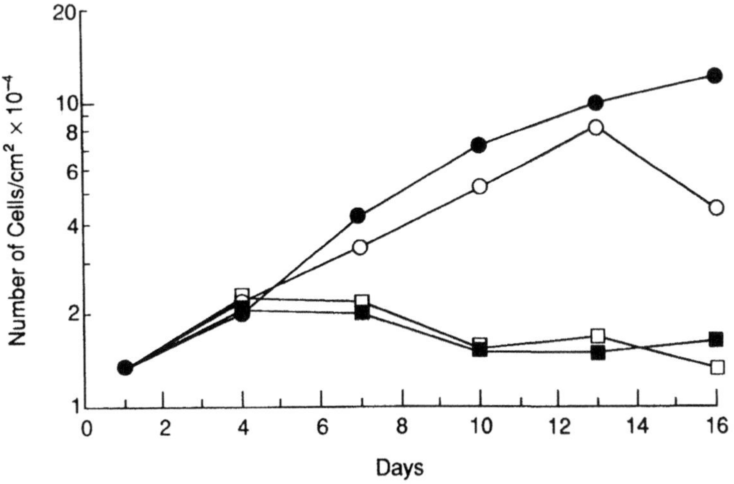

Figure 3. Kinetics of growth of P-B10.BR-*ras* melanocytes. Primary melanocyte cultures transformed with *ras* oncogene were tested after selection (fourth passage) in TAMP-G800 [medium supplemented with TPA (T), dbcAMP (A), melanotropin (M), placental extract (P), and 800 μg/ml G418 (G)]. Test media were AMP (■), TAMP (●), AMP-G400 (□), and TAMP-G400 (400 μg/ml G418) (○). Notice that the melanocytes grew in the presence of the drug G418, which is evidence for expression of the viral-neomycine gene, but not in the absence of TPA, indicating that they did not become independent from melanocyte mitogen.

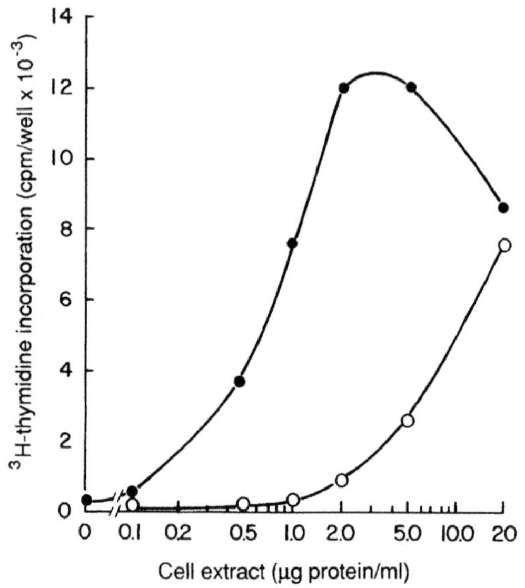

Figure 4. Basic FGF levels in bFGF-transformed melanocytes. Mitogenic response of normal human melanocytes to extract from transfected P-B10.BR (○) and L-B10.BR (●) melanocytes. Extracts were added in PC-1 defined medium plus 1.0 mM dbcAMP for 24 hours to cultures of neonatal melanocytes at the third passage. ^{3}H-thymidine incorporation was performed during the last 3 hours of incubation. Data present the counts per minute for 3 hours and are the average of duplicate wells.

primary murine melanocytes (Figure 3). The failure to transform these cells was probably due to low levels of expression of the transduced genes. The transformed L-B10.BR-bFGF melanocytes expressed approximately 15-fold more biologically active mitogen than the nontransformed P-B10.BR-bFGF melanocytes (Figure 4). Therefore, the ability to acquire growth factor independence is a function of the level of expression of the transduced genes. Immortalized cell lines may be more permissive to transformation because they allow higher expression of foreign genes.

8. Other melanocyte mitogens

Basic FGF belongs to a family of peptides that share approximately 50% homology. This family also includes acidic FGF (aFGF) [72] and the secreted growth factors K-FGF/*hst* (Kaposi's sarcoma growth factor, which is identical with the gene product of human stomach tumor) [73–75], *int*-2 (a cellular gene activated by the integration of mammary tumor virus) [76], FGF-5 [77], FGF-6 [78], and keratinocyte growth factor (KGF) [79]. Some of these factors, i.e., aFGF, K-FGF/*hst*, FGF-5, and FGF-6, but not KGF, are mitogenic toward human melanocytes [27,32] (Table 2). Perhaps significantly, the amino acid simularity between the nonmitogenic KGF and the highly mitogenic FGFs is the lowest [79]. One melanoma out of ten contained amplification of the linked int-2 and K-FGF/hst genes [80], suggesting that growth advantage may be acquired by the action of the two respective gene products.

The mitogenic effect of members from the FGF family on normal human melanocytes in culture is of special importance, because many other mitogens have been tested and proven to be ineffective [27]. They include melanotropin (melanocyte-stimulating hormone), an effective mitogen for murine melanocytes [71]; adrenocorticotropic hormone (ACTH); other pituitary hormones; NGF, EGF, TGF-α, and -β, PDGF; IL-1 and -2; and others [for complete list, see 27]. However, the FGFs are only fully mitogenic in the presence of cAMP stimulators, suggesting the possibility for other natural mitogens. Recent experiments with known and only recently identified factors show that such mitogens indeed exist. Morelli et al. [81] showed

Table 2. Other melanocyte mitogens

Additions	^{3}H-thymidine incorporation (cpm/well/3 hours)
Experiment 1	
hrbFGF	230
dbcAMP	1,290
dbcAMP + hrbFGF	20,200
Cell extracts with dbcAMP with and without anti-bFGF-(1-24)-ab	
NIH 3T3	9,620
NIH 3T3 + anti-bFGF-ab	4,500
FGF-5	24,700
FGF-5 + anti-bFGF-ab	17,300
FGF-6	50,700
FGF-6 + anti-bFGF-ab	47,000
Melanoma YU SIT 1	41,100
Melanoma YU SIT 1 + anti-bFGF-ab	1,100
Experiment 2	
None	700
hrbFGF	3,400
dbcAMP	560
hrbFGF + dbc AMP	24,400
LTC_4	300
LTC_4 + dbc AMP	4,000
LTC_4 + hrbFGF	7,100

Additions were 1 ng/ml hrbFGF (human recombinant basic fibroblast growth factor, Chiron, 1.0 mM dbcAMP (dibutyryladenosine cyclic monophosphate), 100 nM LTC_4 (leukotriene C_4), 100 μg protein/ml cell extract, and 1:100 dilution of anti-bFGF-(1-24)-ab. FGF-5 and FGF-6 are fibroblasts transformed with cDNA clones for the respective growth factor. The cell lines were obtained from Drs. M. Goldfarb and D. Birnbaum, respectively. ^{3}H-thymidine incorporation was performed during the last 3 hours of the 24-hour incubation period. Other details are as in the legend to Table 1. Data are the means of duplicate wells. Notice that anti-bFGF antibodies neutralized only slightly the melanocyte mitogen in extracts from NIH 3T3, FGF-5, and FGF-6 fibroblasts. In contrast, they neutralized all the mitogenic activity in the YU SIT 1 melanoma cell extract, confirming that the melanocyte mitogen in melanomas is bFGF.

that two eicosanoids, the leukotrienes C_4 (LTC_4) and D_4 (LTD_4), stimulate human melanocyte proliferation when supplied in keratinocyte growth medium that contains pituitary extract. Because pituitary extract is rich in bFGF [58], these results suggest that the two leukotrienes acted synergistically with bFGF. Indeed, in our hands, LTC_4 stimulated normal human and murine melanocytes only when supplied with either dbcAMP or bFGF (Table 2). Eicosanoids are inflammatory mediators and therefore might be responsible for postinflammatory hyperpigmentation, as suggested by Morelli et al. [81].

The recently discovered plasminogen-like growth factor (PLGF) [82], which does not belong to the FGF family, is also mitogenic to normal human melanocytes [Halaban, Rubin, and Aaronson, unpublished]. PLGF, isolated and cloned from M426 human embryonic lung fibroblasts, is distinct from keratinocyte growth factor (KGF), cloned from the same cell line [79], as well as from FGF. PLGF stimulates cells of epithelial origin, such as hepatocytes and endothelial cells, but not fibroblasts. It is mitogenic toward melanocytes in a 24-hour stimulation assay when supplied by itself, but its potency is increased synergistically in the presence of dbcAMP or bFGF. PLGF, like bFGF, stimulates a tyrosine-kinase [82]. These results suggest that activation of at least one tyrosine-kinase at the cell surface is needed for full stimulation of melanocytes and that, in vivo, the synergism between bFGF and leukotrienes or PLGF may lead to melanocyte proliferation.

Some melanomas express growth factors other than those from the FGF family, such as PDGF [83], TGF-α [84,85], TGF-β [84], melanoma-derived growth factor (MGSA) [86], IL-1 [87], and as-yet unidentified factors that can stimulate fibroblasts or melanoma cells [84, 88]. Interestingly, cells from some nevi with abnormal karyotype also produced a secreted factor that stimulated a melanoma cell line [88]. However, as indicated before, none of these factors is mitogenic for normal human melanocytes and, in contrast to bFGF [32], no evidence has been provided that their activity is needed for melanoma survival. In addition, normal melanocytes and most melanoma cell lines do not express receptors for PDGF [83] or TGF-α [89], the latter being identical with the EGF receptor. Therefore, the other mitogens produced by melanoma cells may not act as autocrine growth factors, but rather as paracrine factors affecting neighboring cells. Evidence for a paracrine function for TGF-α was suggested by a case report of a patient with acanthosis nigricans secondary to a cutaneous melanoma [85]. In this case, it appeared that TGF-α was secreted by the cutaneous melanoma and, in turn, promoted the development of acanthosis nigricans [85].

9. Concluding remarks and a look to the future

This chapter had as its focus the growth factors and growth factor receptors that are important for the proliferation of normal and malignant melanocytes.

We demonstrated that optimal growth in culture of normal melanocytes requires the synergistic stimulus of two growth factors, one being from the FGF family. Basic FGF was shown to be produced in skin cells in vivo and in vitro. Activation of tyrosine-kinases in melanocytes is probably important for proliferation, because activation of the receptors for two of the known growth factors, bFGF and PLGF, also activates tyrosine kinases. The constitutive activation of one of these receptors, for bFGF, was shown to be required but not sufficient to cause melanomas. Interestingly, the dominant oncogene *Tu* in *Xiphophorus* hybrids was recently identified as a gene encoding a novel receptor tyrosine kinase that is closely related to the EGF receptor [90].

Factors are produced by the environment that either promote or inhibit the growth of transformed melanocytes. Preferential metastasis to the liver was shown to be the result of a melanoma growth factor produced by hepatocytes [91], and the existence of a melanoma inhibitor in certain human myofibroblast lines has also been documented [92]. Interferons, tumor necrosis factor, and TGF-β1 and TGF-β2 are known to restrain normal cell proliferation [93]. Interferons that are used to treat patients with melanomas might be among the inhibitors produced by keratinocytes. One mechanism by which metastatic cells might escape environmental restraints is failure to express the relevant receptors. This was shown in the case of retinoblastoma cell lines that had lost the receptors for TGF-β1 [93]. Future research will probably identify the natural growth promoters and inhibitors for melanomas, and may reveal the mechanism by which melanocytes escape environmental control.

The failure of transduced oncogenes to transform primary melanocytes suggests the existence of suppressing factors in normal cells. The existence of tumor suppressor genes was shown more than a decade ago by the study of hybrids made from malignant and normal cells [94–98]. In hybrids in which the full chromosomal complement of the parental cells was preserved, malignancy was dominantly suppressed [94–98]. Similar results were obtained in hybrids between melanoma cells and fibroblasts that showed, in addition, suppression of differentiated functions [99–101]. Further support for the presence of a melanoma suppressor gene is the frequent deletion or loss of heterozygosity at chromosomal locations 1p 6 and 7 in melanomas and suppression of tumorigenicity by transfer of normal chromosome 6 into melanoma cells [54,114]. It appears that this region contains a dysplastic nevus/malignant melanoma susceptibility gene [102], although more recent studies have not confirmed this observation [115,116]. The cloning and characterization of the retinoblastoma susceptibility gene and the demonstration that this gene acts as a tumor suppressor is one of the most exciting events in the field of tumor biology [103–106]. The identification of such genes in melanocytes will further clarify the mechanism by which normal melanocytes resist becoming malignant.

Knowledge of the importance of bFGF receptor activity in melanomas may be used to devise new drugs for therapy. The drugs can be directed toward blocking the binding of FGF to the receptor or to inhibit the tyrosine-kinase activity. There is a precedence for such an approach. For example, low molecular weight tyrphostins have been developed that inhibit the tyrosine-kinase of the EGF receptor more effectively than that of the insulin receptor by three orders of magnitude [102]. These substances inhibit the proliferation in culture of a carcinoma cell line expressing high levels of EGF receptors [107]. The melanocyte growth factors can also be covalently linked to a drug. The efficacy of such drugs for melanocytes would be determined by the expression of the receptors in vivo.

Acknowledgements

I thank Drs. Gisela Moellmann and Jean Bolognia for critically reading the manuscript and for helpful suggestions, Dr.A.B.Lerner for support, and Sarah Straight and Jack Schreiber for technical help.

This work was supported by Public Health Service Grants 1 R29 CA44542 and 5 RO1 CA 04679 and 5 PO1 AR25252.

References

1. Todaro, G.J., DeLarco, J.E. (1978) Growth factors produced by sarcoma virus-transformed cells. Cancer Res. 38:4147–4154.
2. Sporn, M.B., Roberts, A.B. (1987) Autocrine growth factors and cancer. Nature 313: 745–747.
3. Keski-Oja, J., Lyons, R.M., Moses, H.L. (1987) Immunodetection and modulation of cellular growth with antibodies against native transforming growth factor-β. Cancer Res. 47:6451–6458.
4. Huang, S.S., Huang, J.S., Deuel, T.F. (1984) Transforming protein of simian sarcoma virus stimulates autocrine growth of SSV-transformed cells through PDGF cell-surface receptors. Cell 39:79–87.
5. Pantaziz, P., Lanfrancone, L., Pelicci, P.G., Dalla-Favera, R., Antoniades, H.N. (1986) Human leukemia cells synthesize and secrete proteins related to platelet-derived growth factor. Proc. Natl. Acad. Sci. USA 83:5526–5530.
6. Cozzolino, F., Rubartelli, A., Aldinucci, D., Sitia, R., Torcia, M., Shaw, A., Di Guglielmo, R. (1989) Interleukin 1 as an autocrine growth factor for acute myeloid leukemia cells. Proc. Natl. Acad. Sci. USA 86:2369–2373.
7. Duprez, V., Lenoir, G., Dautry-Varsat, A. (1985) Autocrine growth stimulation of a human T-cell lymphoma line by interleukin 2. Proc. Natl. Acad. Sci. USA 82:6932–6936.
8. Chen, S.J., Holbrook, N.J., Mitchell, K.F., Vallone, C.A., Greengard, J.S., Crabtree, G.R., Lin, Y. (1985) A viral long terminal repeat in the interleukin 2 gene of a cell line that constitutively produces interleukin 2. Proc. Natl. Acad. Sci. USA 82:7284–7288.
9. Ymer, S., Tucker, W.Q.J., Sanderson, C.J., Hapel, A.J., Campbell, H.D., Young, I.G. (1985) Constitutive synthesis of interleukin-3 by leukemia cell line WEHI-3B is due to retroviral insertion near the gene. Nature 317:255–258.
10. Andrejauskas, E., Moroni, C. (1989) Reversible abrogation of IL-3 dependence by an inducible H-*ras* oncogene. EMBO J. 8:2575–2581.
11. Stern, D.F., Hare, D.L., Cecchini, M.A., Weinberg, R.A. (1987) Construction of a novel oncogene based on synthetic sequences encoding epidermal growth factor. Science 235:321–324.

12. Kacinski, B.M., Carter, D., Mittal, K., Kohorn, E.I., Bloodgood, S., Donahue, J., Donofrio, L., Edwards, R., Schwartz, P.E., Chambers, J.T., Chambers, S.K. (1988) High level expression of *fms* proto-oncogene mRNA is observed in clinically aggressive human endometrial adenocarcinomas. Int. J. Rad. Onc. Biol. Phys. 15:823–829.
13. Bargmann, C.I., Hung, M-C., Weinberg, R.A. (1986) Multiple independent activations of the *neu* oncogene by a point mutation altering the transmembrane domain of p185. Cell 45:649–657.
14. Di Fiore, P.P., Pierce, J.H., Kraus, M.H., Segatto, O., King, C.R., Aaronson, S.A. (1987) *erbB*-2 is a potent oncogene when overexpressed in NIH/3T3 cells. Science 237:178–182.
15. Di Fiore, P.P., Pierce, J.H., Fleming, T.P., Hazan, R., Ullrich, A., King, CR., Schlessinger, J., Aaronson, S.A. (1987) Overexpression of the human EGF receptor confers and EGF-dependent transformed phenotype to NIH 3T3 cells. Cell 51:1063–1070.
16. Velu, T.J., Beguinot, L, Vass, W.C., Willingham, M.C., Merlino, G.T., Pastan, I., Lowy, D.R. (1987) Epidermal growth factor-dependent transformation by a human EGF receptor proto-oncogene. Science 238:1408–1410.
17. Kraus, M.H., Issing, W., Miki, T., Popescu, N.C., Aaronson, S.A. (1989) Isolation and characterization of *ERBB3*, a third member of the *ERBB*/epidermal growth factor receptor family: Evidence for overexpression in a subset of human mammary tumors. Proc. Natl. Acad. Sci. USA 86:9193–9197.
18. Bishop, J.M. (1983) Cellular oncogenes and retroviruses. Ann. Rev. Biochem. 52:301–354.
19. Downward, J., Yarden, Y., Mayes, E., Scrace, G., Totty, N., Stockwell, P., Ullrich, A., Schlessinger, J., Waterfield, M.D. (1984) Close similarity of epidermal growth factor receptor and v-*erb*-B oncogene protein sequences. Nature 307:521–527.
20. Hampe, A., Gohet, M., Sherr, C.J., Galibert, F. (1984) Nucleotide sequence of the feline retroviral oncogene v-*fms* shows unexpected homology with oncogenes controlling tyrosine-specific protein kinases. Proc. Natl. Acad. Sci. USA 81:85–89.
21. Coussens, L., Yang-Feng, T.L., Liao, Y.-C., Chen, E., Gray, A., McGrath, J., Seeburg, P.H., Liberman, T.A., Schlessinger, J., Francke, U., Levinson, A., Ullrich, A. (1985) Tyrosine kinase receptor with extensive homology to EGF receptor shares chromosomal location with *neu* oncogene. Science 230:1132–1139.
22. Green S., Walter, P., Kumar, V., Krust, A., Bornert, J.-M., Argos, P., Chambon, P. (1986) Human oestrogen receptor cDNA: Sequence, expression and homology to v-*erb*-A. Nature 320:134–139.
23. Sap, J., Muñoz, A., Damm, K., Goldberg, Y., Ghysdael, J., Leutz, A., Beug, H., Vennström, B. (1986) The c-*erb*-A protein is a high-affinity receptor for thyroid hormone. Nature 324:635–640.
24. Weinberger, C, Thompson, C.C., Ong, E.S., Lebo, R., Gruol, D.J., Evans, R.M. (1986) The c-*erb*-A gene encodes a thyroid hormone receptor. Nature 324:641–646.
25. Roussel, M.R., Dull, T.J., Rettenmeier, C.W., Ralph, P.W., Ullrich, A., Sherr, C.J. (1987) Transforming potential of the c-*fms* proto-oncogene (CSF-1 receptor). Nature 325:549–552.
26. Wells, A., Bishop, J.M. (1988) Genetic determinants of neoplastic transformation by the retroviral oncogene v-*erbB*. Proc. Natl. Acad. Sci. USA 85:7597–7601.
27. Halaban, R. (1988) Responses of cultured melanocytes to defined growth factors. Pigment Cell Res. 1:18–26.
28. Eisinger, M., Marko, O., (1982) Selective proliferation of normal human melanocytes in vitro in the presence of phorbol ester and cholera toxin. Proc. Natl. Acad. Sci. USA 79:2018–2022.
29. Eisinger, O., Marko, O., Weinstein, I.B. (1983) Stimulation of growth of human melanocytes by tumor promoters. Carcinogenesis 4:779–781.
30. Halaban, R., Ghosh, S., Duray, P., Kirkwood, J.M., Lerner, A.B. (1986) Human melanocytes cultured from nevi and melanomas. J. Invest. Dermatol. 87:95–101.
31. Halaban, R., Ghosh, S., Baird, A. (1987) bFGF is the putative natural growth factor for human melanocytes. In Vitro Cell Dev. Biol. 23:47–52.

32. Halaban, R., Kwon, B.S., Ghosh, S., Delli Bovi, P., Baird, A. (1988) bFGF as an autocrine growth factor for human melanomas. Oncogene Res. 3:177–186.
33. Halaban, R., Langdon, R., Birchall, N., Cuono, C., Baird, A., Scott, G., Moellmann, G., McGuire, J. (1988) Basic fibroblast growth factor of keratinocytes is a natural mitogen for normal human melanocytes. J Cell Biol 107:1611–1619.
34. Eisinger, M., Marko, O., Ogata, S.-L., Old, L.J. (1985) Growth regulation of human melanocytes: Mitogenic factors in extracts of melanoma, astrocytoma, and fibroblast cell lines. Science 229:984–986.
35. Lobb, R., Sasse, J., Sullivan, R., Shing, Y., D'Amore, P., Jacobs, J., Klagsbrun, M. (1986) Purification and characterization of heparin-binding endothelial cell growth factors. J. Biol. Chem. 261:1924–1926.
36. Moscatelli, D., Presta, M., Joseph-Silverstein, J., Rifkin, D.B. (1986) Both normal and tumor cells produce basic fibroblast growth factor. J. Cell. Physiol. 129:273–276.
37. Ogata, S., Furuhashi, Y., Eisinger, M. (1987) Growth stimulation of human melanocytes: Identification and characterization of melanoma-derived growth factor (M-McGF). Biochem. Biophys. Res. Commun. 146:1204–1211.
38. Becker, D., Meier, C.B., Herlyn, M. (1989) Proliferation of human malignant melanomas is inhibited by antisense oligodeoxynucleotides targeted against basic fibroblast growth factor. EMBO J. 8:3685–3691.
39. Kirchheimer, J.C., Wojta, J., Christ, G., Binder, B.R. (1989) Functional inhibition of endogenously produced urokinase decreases cell proliferation in a human melanoma cell line. Proc. Natl. Acad. Sci. USA 86:5424–5428.
40. Sato, Y., Rifkin, D.B. (1988) Autocrine activities of basic fibroblast growth factor: Regulation of endothelial cell movement, plasminogen activator synthesis and DNA synthesis. J. Cell Biol. 107:1199–1205.
41. Browder, T.M., Dunbar, C.E., Nienhuis, A.W. (1989) Private and public autocrine loops in neoplastic cells. Cancer Cells 1:9–17.
42. Abraham, J.A., Mergia, A., Whang, J.L., Tumolo, A., Friedman, J., Hjerrild, K.A., Gospodarowicz, D., Fiddes, J.C. (1986) Nucleotide sequence of a bovine clone encoding the angiogenic protein, basic fibroblast growth factor. Science 233:545–548.
43. Abraham, J.A., Whang, J.L., Tumolo, A., Mergia, A., Friedman, J., Gospodarowicz, D., Fiddes, J.C. (1986) Human basic fibroblast growth factor: Nucleotide sequence and genomic organization. EMBO J. 5:2523–2528.
44. Jeanny, J.-C., Fayein, N., Moenner, M., Chavallier, B., Barritault, D., Courtois, Y. (1987) Specific fixation of bovine brain and retinal acidic and basic fibroblast growth factors to mouse embryonic eye basement membranes. Exp. Cell. Res. 171:63–75.
45. Vlodavsky, I., Folkman, J., Sullivan, R., Fridman, R., Ishai-Michaeli, R., Sasse, J., Klagsbrun, M. (1987) Endothelial cell-derived basic fibroblast growth factor: Synthesis and decomposition into subendothelial extracellular matrix. Proc. Natl. Acad. Sci. USA 84:2292–2296.
46. Huang, J.S., Huang, S.S., Deuel, T.F. (1984) Transforming protein of simian sarcoma virus stimulates autocrine growth of SSV-transformed cells through PDGF cell-surface receptors. Cell 39:79–87.
47. Hannink, M., Donoghue, D.J. (1986) Biosynthesis of the v-*sis* gene products: Signal sequence cleavage, glycosylation, and proteolytic processing. Mol. Cell. Biol. 6:1343–1348.
48. Yeh, H.-J., Pierce, G.F., Deuel, T.F. (1987) Ultrastructural localization of a platelet-derived growth factor/v-*sis*-related protein(s) in cytoplasm and nucleus of simian sarcoma virus-transformed cells. Proc. Natl. Acad. Sci. USA 84:2317–2321.
49. Lang, R.A., Metcalf, D., Gough, N.M., Dunn, A.R., Gonda, T.J. (1985) Expression of a hemopoietic growth factor-dependent cell line results in autonomous growth and tumorigenicity. Cell 43:531–542.
50. Laker, C., Stocking, C., Bergholz, U., Hess, N., De Lamarter, J.F., Ostertag, W. (1987) Autocrine stimulation after transfer of the granulocyte/macrophage colony-stimulating factor gene and autonomous growth are distinct but interdependent steps in the oncogenic

pathway. Proc. Natl. Acad. Sci. USA 84:8458–8462.
51. Browder, T.M., Abrams, J.S., Wong , P.M.C., Nienhuis, A.W. (1989) Mechanism of autocrine stimulation in hematopoietic cells producing interleukin-3 after retrovirus-mediated gene transfer. Mol. Cell. Biol. 9:204–213.
52. Dotto, G., Ghosh S., Moellmann G., Lerner A.B., Halaban R. (1989) Transformation of melanocytes with basic fibroblast growth factor cDNA and oncogenes and selective suppression of the transformed phenotype in a reconstituted cutaneous environment. J. Cell. Biol. 109:3115–3128.
53. Mergia, A., Eddy, R., Abraham, J.A., Fiddes, J.C., Shows, T.B. (1986) The genes for basic and acidic fibroblast growth factors are on different human chromosomes. Biochem. Biophys. Res. Commun. 138:644–651.
54. Balaban, G., Herlyn, M., Guerry IV, D., Bartolo, R., Koprowski, H., Clark, W.H., Nowell, P.C. (1984) Cytogenetics of human malignant melanoma and premalignant lesions. Cancer Genet. Cytogenet. 11:429–439.
55. Dracopoli, N.C., Houghton, A.N., Old, L.J. (1985) Loss of polymorphic restriction fragments in malignant melanoma: Implications for tumor heterogeneity. Proc. Natl. Acad. Sci. USA 82:1470–1474.
56. Cowan, J.M., Halaban, R., Francke, U. (1988) Cytogenetic analysis of melanocytes from premalignant nevi and melanomas. J. Natl. Cancer Inst. 80:1159–1164; Cancer Genet. Cytogenet 20:255–261.
57. Theillet, C., Le Roy, X., De Lapeyrière, O., Grosgeorges, J., Adnane, J., Raynaud, S.D., Simony-Lafontaine, J., Goldfarb, M., Escot, C., Birnbaum, D., Gaudray, P. (1989) Amplification of FGF-related genes in human tumors: Possible involvement of HST in breast carcinomas. Oncogene 4:915–922.
58. Rifkin, D.B., Moscatelli, D. (1989) Recent developments in the cell biology of basic fibroblast growth factor. J. Cell. Biol. 109:1–6.
59. Huang, S.S., Huang, J.S. (1986) Association of bovine brain-derived growth factor receptor with protein tyrosine kinase activity. J. Biol. Chem. 261:9568–9571.
60. Coughlin, S.R., Barr, P.J., Cousens, L.S., Fretto, L.J., Williams, L.T. (1988) Acidic and basic fibroblast growth factors stimulate tyrosine kinase activity in vivo. J. Biol. Chem. 263:988–993.
61. Lee, P.L., Johnson, D.E., Cousens, L.S., Fried, V.A., Williams, L.T. (1989) Purification and complementary DNA cloning of a receptor for basic fibroblast growth factor. Science 245:57–60.
62. Ruta, M., Burgess, W., Givol, D., Epstein, J., Neiger, N., Kaplow, J., Crumley, G., Dionne, C., Jaye, M, Schlessinger, J. (1989) Receptor for acidic fibroblast growth factor is related to the tyrosine kinase encoded by the *fms*-like gene (FLG). Proc. Natl. Acad. Sci. USA 86:8722–8726.
63. Greene, M.H., Clark, W.H. Jr., Tucker, M.A., Kraemer, K.H., Elder, D.E., Fraser, M.C. (1985) High risk of malignant melanoma in melanoma-prone families with dysplastic nevi. Ann. Intern. Med. 102:458–465.
64. Halaban, R., Pomerantz, S.H., Marshall, S., Lambert, D.T., Lerner, A.B. (1983) Regulation of tyrosinase in human melanocytes grown in culture. J. Cell Biol. 97:480–488.
65. Halaban, R., Pomerantz, S.H., Marshall, S., Lerner, A.B. (1984) Tyrosinase activity and abundance in Cloudman melanoma cells. Arch. Biochem. Biophys. 230:383–387.
66. Kwon, B.S., Halaban, R., Kim, G.S., Usack, L., Pomerantz, S., Haq, A.K. (1987) A melanocyte-specific cDNA clone whose expression is inducible by melanotropin and isobutylmethyl xanthine. Molec. Biol. Med. 4:339–355.
67. Kwon, B.S., Wakulchik, M., Haq, A.K., Halaban, R., Kestler, D. (1988) Sequence analysis of murine tyrosinase cDNA and the effect of melanotropin on its gene expression. Biochem. Biophys. Res. Commun. 153:1301–1309.
68. Dotto, GP., O'Connell, J., Patskan, G., Conti, C. Ariza, A., Slaga, T. (1989) Malignant progression of papilloma-derived keratinocytes: Differential effects of the *ras*, *neu*, and *p53* oncogenes. Mol. Carcinogen. 1:171–179.

69. Finlay, C.A., Hinds, P.W., Levine, A.J. (1989) The p53 proto-oncogene can act as a suppressor of transformation. Cell 57:1083–1093.
70. Halaban, R. Growth regulation in normal and malignant melanocytes. (1990) In Ferrone, S., ed., Human Melanoma. Springer-Verlag, Berlin, 1990, pp. 3–14.
71. Tamura, A., Halaban, R., Moellmann, G., Cowan, J.M., Lerner, M.R., Lerner, A.B. (1987) Normal murine melanocytes in culture. In Vitro Cell Dev. Biol. 23:519–522.
72. Jaye, M., Howk, J.R., Burgess, W., Ricca, G.A., Chiu, I.-M., Ravera, M.W., O'Brien, S.J., Modi, W.S., Maciag, T., Drohan, W.N. (1986) Human endothelial cell growth factor: Cloning nucleotide sequence, and chromosome localization. Science 233:541–545.
73. Delli Bovi, P., Basilico, C. (1987) Isolation of a rearranged human transforming gene following transfection of Kaposi sarcoma DNA. Proc. Natl. Acad. Sci. USA 84:5660–5664.
74. Delli Bovi, P., Curatola, A.M., Kern, F.G., Creco, A., Ittmann, M., Basilico, C. (1987) An oncogene isolated by transfection of Kaposi's sarcoma DNA encodes a growth factor that is a member of the FGF family. Cell 50:729–737.
75. Taira, M., Yoshida, T., Miyagawa, K., Sakamoto, H., Terada, M., Sugimura, T. (1987) cDNA sequence of human transforming gene *hst* and identification of the coding sequence required for transforming activity. Proc. Natl. Acad. Sci. USA 84:2980–2984.
76. Dickson, C., Peters, G. (1987) Potential oncogene product related to growth factors. Nature (London) 326:833.
77. Zhan, X., Bates, B. Hu, X., Goldfarb, M. (1988) The human FGF-5 oncogene encodes a novel protein related to fibroblast growth factors. Mol. Cell Biol. 8:3487–3495.
78. Marics, I., Adelaide, J., Raybaud, F., Mattei, M.-G., Coulier, F., Planche, J., de Lapeyriere, O., Birnbaum, D. (1989) Characterization of the *HST*-related FGF.6 gene, a new member of the fibroblast growth factor family. Oncogene 4:335–340.
79. Finch, P.W., Rubin, J.S., Miki, T., Ron, D., Aaronson, S.A. (1989) Human KGF is FGF-related with properties of a paracrine effector of epithelial cell growth. Science 245:752–755.
80. Adelaide, J., Mattei, M.-G., Marics, I., Raybaud, F., Planche, J., De Lapeyriere, O., Birnbaum, D. (1988) Chromosomal localization of the *hst* oncogene and its co-amplification with the *int*.2 oncogene in human melanoma. Oncogene 2:413–416.
81. Morelli, J.G., Yohn, J.J., Lyons, M.B., Murphy, R.C., Norris D.A. (1989) Leukotrienes C_4 and D_4 as potent mitogens for cultured human neonatal melanocytes. J. Invest. Dermatol. 93:719–722.
82. Rubin, F.S., Chan, A. M.-L., Bottaro, D.P., Wilson, H.B., Taylor, W.G., Cech, A.C., Hirschfeld, D.W., Wong, J., Miki, T., Finch, P.W., Aaronson, S.A. (1990) A broad spectrum human lung fibroblast-derived mitogen is homologous to hepatocyte growth factor. Proc. Natl. Acad. Sci. USA, in press.
83. Westermark, B., Johnsson, A., Paulsson, Y., Betscholtz, C., Heldin, C.-H., Herlyn, M., Rodeck, U., Koprowski, H. (1986) Human melanoma cell lines of primary and metastatic origin express the genes encoding the chains of platelet-derived growth factor (PDGF) and produce PDGF-like growth factor. Proc. Natl. Acad. Sci. USA 83:7197–7200.
84. De-Larco, J.E., Pigott, D.A., Lazarus, J.A. (1985) Ectopic peptides released by a human melanoma cell line that modulate the transformed phenotype. Proc. Natl. Acad. Sci. USA 82:5015–5019.
85. Ellis, D.L., Kafka, S.P., Chow, J.C., Nanney, L.B., Inman, W.H., McGadden, M.E., King, L.E. Jr. (1987) Melanoma, growth factors, acanthosis nigricans, the sign of Leser-Trelat, and multiple acrochordons: A possible role for alpha-transforming growth factor in cutaneous paraneoplastic syndromes. N. Engl. J. Med. 317:1582–1587.
86. Richmond, A., Balentien, E., Thomas, H.G., Flaggs, G., Barton, D.E., Spiess, J., Bordoni, R., Francke, U, Derynck, R. (1988) Molecular characterization and chromosomal mapping of melanoma growth stimulatory activity, a growth factor structurally related to β-thromboglobulin. EMBO J. 7:2025–2033.
87. Köck, A., Schwarz, T., Urbanski, A., Peng, Z., Vetterlein, M., Micksche, M., Ansel, J.C., Kung, H.F., Luger, T.A. (1989) Expression and release of interleukin-1 by different

human melanoma cell lines. J. Natl. Cancer Inst. 81:36–42.
88. Richmood, A., Fine, R., Murray, D., Lawson, D.H., Priest, J.H. (1986) Growth factor and cytogenetic abnormalities in cultured nevi and malignant melanomas. J. Invest. Dermatol. 86:295–302.
89. Real, F.X., Retting, W.G., Chesa, P.G., Melamed, M.R., Old, L.R., Mendelsohn, J. (1986) Expression of epidermal growth factor receptor in human cultured cells and tissues: Relationship to cell lineage and stage of differentiation. Cancer Res. 46:4726–4731.
90. Wittbrodt, J., Adam, D., Malitschek, B. Mäueler, W., Raulf, F., Telling, A., Robertson, S.M., Schartl, M. (1989) Novel putative receptor tyrosine kinase encoded by the melanoma-inducing *Tu* locus in *Xiphophorus*. Nature 341:415–421.
91. Sargent, N.S., Oestreicher, M., Haidvogl, H., Madnick, H.M., Burger, M.M. (1988) Growth regulation of cancer metastases by their host organ. Proc. Natl. Acad. Si. USA 85:7251–7255.
92. Wu, K.-F., Pope, J.H., Ellem, K.A.O. (1985) Inhibition of growth of certain human tumour cell lines by a factor derived from human fibroblast-like cell lines. I. Demonstration by mixed culture and use of cell washings. Int. J. Cancer 35:477–482.
93. Kimchi, A., Wang, X.-F., Weinberg, R., Cheifetz, S., Massagué, J. (1988) Absence of TGF-β receptors and growth inhibitory responses in retinoblastoma cells. Science 240: 196–199.
94. Wiener, F., Fenyö, E.M., Klein, G. (1972) Fusion of tumor cells with host cells. Nature (London) 238:155–159.
95. Wiener, F., Klein, G., Harris, H. (1974) The analysis of malignancy by cell fusion. J. Cell Sci. 15:177–183.
96. Stanbridge, E.J., Der, C. J., Doersen, C.-J., Nishimi, R. Y., Peehl, D.M., Weissman, B.E., Wilkinson, J.E. (1982) Human cell hybrids: Analysis of transformation and tumorigenicity. Science 215:252–259.
97. Klein, G. (1987) The approaching era of the tumor suppressor genes. Science 238:1539–1545.
98. Sager, R. (1989) Tumor suppressor genes: The puzzle and the promise. Science 246: 1406–1412.
99. Fougère, C., Ruiz, F., Ephrussi, B. (1972) Gene dosage dependence of pigment synthesis in melanoma x fibroblast hybrids. Proc. Natl. Acad. Sci USA 69:330–334.
100. Straus, D.S., Jonasson, J., Harris, H. (1976) Growth in vitro of tumor cell x fibroblast hybrids in which malignancy is suppressed. J. Cell Sci. 25:73–86.
101. Halaban, R., Moellmann, G., Godawska, E., Eisenstadt, J. (1980) Pigmentation and tumorigenicity of reconstituted, cybrid and hybrid mouse cells. Exp. Cell Res. 130:427–435.
102. Bale, S.J., Dracopoli, N.C., Tucker, M.A., Clark, W.H. Jr., Fraser, M.C., Stranger, B.Z., Green, P., Donis-Keller, H., Housman, D.E., Greene, M.H. (1989) Mapping the gene for hereditary cutaneous malignant melanoma-dysplastic nevus to chromosome 1p. N. Engl. J. Med. 320:1376–1372.
103. Lee, W.-H., Bookstein, R., Hong, F., Young, L.-J., Shew, J.-Y., Lee, E.Y.-H.P. (1987) Human retinoblastoma susceptibility gene: Cloning, identification, and sequence. Science 235:1394–1399.
104. Huang, H.-J.S., Yee, J.-K., Shew, H.-Y., Chen, P.-L., Bookstein, R., Friedmann, T., Lee, E.Y.-H.P., Lee, W.-H. (1988) Suppression of the neoplastic phenotype by replacement of the RB gene in human cancer cells. Science 242:1563–1566.
105. Hong, F.D., Huang, H.-J.S., To, H., Young, L.-J.S. Oro, A., Bookstein, R., Lee, E.Y.-H.P., Lee, W.-H. (1989) Structure of the human retinoblastoma gene. Proc. Natl. Acad. Sci. USA 86:5502–5506.
106. Bernards, R., Schackleford, G.M., Gerber, M.R., Horowitz, J.M., Friend, S.H., Schartl, M., Bogenman, E., Rapaport, J.M., McGee, T., Dryja, T.P., Weinberg, R.A. (1989) Structure and expression of the murine retinoblastoma gene and characterization of its encoded protein. Proc. Natl. Acad. Sci. USA 86:6474–6478.
107. Yaish, P., Gazit, A., Gilon, C., Levitzki, A. (1988) Blocking of EGF-dependent cell

proliferation by EGF receptor kinase inhibitors. Science 242:933–935.

108. Mansukhani, A., Moscatelli, D., Talarico, D., Levytska, V., Basilico, C. (1990) A murine fibroblast growth factor (FGF) receptor expressed in CHO cells is activated by basic FGF and Kaposi FGF. Proc. Natl. Acad. Sci. USA 87:4378–4382.
109. Dionne, C.A., Crumley, G., Bellot, F., Kaplow, J.M., Searfoss, G., Ruta, M., Burgess, W.H., Jaye, M., Schlessinger, J. (1990) Cloning and expression of two distinct high-affinity receptors cross-reacting with acidic and basic fibroblast growth factors. EMBO J 9: 2685–2692.
110. Johnson, D.E., Lee, P.L., Lu, J., Williams, L.T. (1990) Diverse forms of a receptor for acidic and basic fibroblast growth factors. Mol. Cell. Biol. 10:4728–4736.
111. Hattori, Y., Odagiri, H., Nakatani, H., Miyagawa, K., Naito, K., Sakamoto, H., Katoh, O., Yoshida, T., Sugimura, T., Terada, M. (1990) K-*sam*, an amplified gene in stomach cancer, is a member of the heparin-binding growth factor receptor genes. Proc. Natl. Acad. Sci. USA 87:5983–5987.
112. Tessler, S., Neufeld, G. (1990) Basic fibroblast growth factor (bFGF) accumulates in the nuclei of various bFGF producing cell types. J. Cell. Physiol., in press.
113. Scott, G., Stoler, M., Sarkar, S., Halaban, R. (1990) Localization of basic fibroblast growth factor mRNA in melanocytic lesions by *in situ* hybridization. J. Invest. Dermatol., in press.
114. Trent, J., Stanbridge, E.J., McBride, H.L., Meese, E.U., Casey, G., Araujo, D.E., Witkowski, C.M., Nagle, R.B. (1990) Tumorigenicity in human melanoma cell lines controlled by introduction of human chromosome 6. Science 247:568–571.
115. Gruis, N.A., Bergman, W., Frants, R.R. (1990) Locus for susceptibility to melanoma on chromosome 1p. New Engl. J. Med. 322:853–854.
116. Cannon-Albright, L.A., Goldgar, D.E., Wright, E.C., Turco, A., Jost, M., Meyer L.J. (1990) Evidence against the reported linkage of the cutaneous melanoma-dysplastic nevus syndrome locus to chromosome 1p36. Am. J. Hum. Genet. 46:918–921.

3. Cytokines and Human Malignant Melanoma Immuno- and Growth-Regulatory Peptides in Melanoma Biology

A. Köck, T. Schwarz, M. Micksche, and T.A. Luger

1. Introduction

The incidence of malignant melanoma has dramatically increased worldwide during the last decade, and no effective treatment modalities exist for advanced stages of this malignancy [1]. Therefore new therapeutic strategies need to be developed [2]. Accordingly, it seems to be of great importance to elucidate the biology of this fatal skin disease in order to discover new treatment modalities that interfere with the growth behavior of malignant melanoma.

Evidence exists that immunological factors play an essential role in the biological behavior and therefore in the clinical course of malignant melanoma. The phenomenon of spontaneous tumor regression [3], as well as the occurrence of metastatic lesions, even 10 years after initial radical surgery of the primary tumor, emphasize the importance of immune mechanisms in the control of this disease. Furthermore, dense lymphocytic infiltrates detected in many, but not all, primary and metastatic nodules, and the recent finding that these tumor infiltrating lymphocytes can be activated to potent killer cells for therapeutic use supports the notion that immune reactions are actively involved in the defense mechanisms against malignant melanoma [4].

The question of whether soluble mediators released by melanoma cells influence the immune reactions or whether tumor cell derived growth factors influence the clinical behavior of this disease has not yet been clearly elucidated. In the present review, we will focus on cytokines and growth factors produced by melanoma cells and their importance for growth behavior of human malignant melanoma, both in vitro and in vivo. Furthermore, the potential clinical use of recombinant cytokines and growth factors will briefly be discussed.

2. General aspects of cytokines

Cytokines are multifunctional and multitargeted soluble factors that play an important role in the mediation of inflammatory and immunologic reactions

L. Nathanson (ed.), MELANOMA RESEARCH: GENETICS, GROWTH FACTORS, METASTASES, AND ANTIGENS.

[5]. There is ample evidence that most nucleated cells exhibit the capacity to release at least some of these mediators [6]. Cytokines may not only function locally at the site of release, but may also gain access to the circulation and thus cause systemic effects, e.g., modulation of immunity and inflammation, either in a stimulating or depressing manner [7]. Since several transformed or neoplastic cells have turned out as potent cellular sources for cytokines, the question of whether melanoma cells release such mediators and how that relates to the immune response has raised great interest within the last years.

Cytokines or peptide regulatory factors are (glyco) proteins that bind to specific receptors and influence activation, proliferation, and differentiation of both immune and nomimmune cells. Originally these hormonelike substances were thought to be exclusively released by lymphocytes, and their effect was thought to be confined only to immune cells, therefore the term *lymphokines* was used [5]. However, it turned out that, not only other immune cells, such as macrophages or granulocytes, but also many other cells, such as fibroblasts, endothelial cells, and epithelial cells, including keratinocytes and stroma cells, exhibit the capacity to release these regulatory factors [8]. They originally were described according to their biological activity detected in cell culture supernatants. Since most cells simultaneously release several factors that can sometimes affect the same target cell in a stimulating or suppressive manner, it turned out to be difficult to isolate these mediators by biological and biochemical methods. Recently, due to new molecular biology techniques, great progress has been achieved in identifying the structure and the gene of most cytokines. Moreover, several cytokines are now produced by recombinant DNA techniques and can be provided in sufficient quantities for use as biological response modifiers (BRM) in clinical trials.

All cytokines exhibit pleiotropic biological activities affecting the same or different target cells that express specific cell membrane receptors. In addition, several of these factors can regulate their own release and/or that of other mediators as well as cytokine receptor expression. Accordingly, there is strong evidence for a network of interacting cytokines maintaining a proper balance of immune reactions under physiological conditions. Pathological events, however, may induce the release of some mediators, which by themselves stimulate or inhibit the production of other factors. The activation of this cytokine cascade might be an initial event in pathological reactions and in the manifestation of clinical symptoms.

Due to their multiple and overlapping biological activities, it is impossible to classify cytokines according to simple schemes. The interferons (IFNα, β, γ), interleukin (IL)-6, and tumor necrosis factor (TNF) were originally categorized in the group of factors with antiviral activity [9–11]. Recently, however, it turned out that the antiviral effect of IL-6 and TNF may be indirect due to the induction of the release of IFN [12]. In addition, IL-1, IL-6, and TNF may play an important role in the mediation of inflammatory reactions and of an acute-phase response [13–15]. Colony stimulating factors

(CSF) induce the differentiation and proliferation of both bone marrow and of mature blood cells and include interleukin-3 (IL-3), granulocyte/macrophage-CSF (GM-CSF), granulocyte-CSF (G-CSF), and macrophage-CSF (M-CSF) [16]. Primarily T-cell-derived factors are IL-2, IL-4, IL-5, and IL-7, and these factors play an important role in T- and B-cell activation [17]. Recently, a group of related chemoattractant factors, mainly activating neutrophils, has been characterized and collectively called IL-8 [18]. Currently increasing interest has been raised by another group of mediators, the suppressor factors or anti-cytokines. These, at the moment, are not very well characterized factors that inhibit the biological activities of several cytokines, thus functioning in an antagonistic way [19]. Growth factors that mainly control cell proliferation include epidermal growth factor (EGF), transforming growth factor (TGF), fibroblast growth factor (FGF), and platelet derived growth factor (PDGF) [20]. These factors play an important role in the induction and maintenance of malignant cell growth.

The following chapters will focus on cytokines, such as IL-1, IL-6, and growth factors that are known to be produced by melanoma cells (Table 1) or melanocytes, and/or whose release, even if by other cells, may have important implications in the pathogenesis and biological behavior of malignant melanoma.

3. Immunoregulatory cytokines produced by melanoma cells

3.1. *Interleukin-1 (IL-1)*

Interleukin-1 originally has been described as a lymphocyte activating factor that is released only by monocytes [21]. Later it became evident that a variety of previously described soluble products exhibited the same biological as well as biochemical characteristics, and therefore the term *interleukin-1* was introduced [22]. Moreover, it turned out that, in addition to monocytes, a variety of cells, including endothelial cells and keratinocytes, can produce this multifunctional mediator [23,24]. Both in the human and murine systems, two different forms of IL-1 — IL-1α and IL-1β — have been found [25–27]. Although there is only 30% amino acid homology between the IL-1 subtypes, both share the same spectrum of biological activities and bind to the same receptor with equal affinity [25]. Both IL-1 forms are produced as 31-kD precursor peptides, which subsequently, through the action of specific proteases, have to be cleaved into the 17-kD molecules. Whereas both IL-1α peptides are biologically active, the 31-kD IL-1β precursor lacks any biological activity [28]. In contrast to macrophages that produce mainly IL-1β, the major IL-1 species released by keratinocytes is IL-1α [28]. IL-1 is a multifunctional cytokine, and one of its first functions described was its capacity to activate lymphocytes and to stimulate the proliferation of thymocytes in response to mitogens [21,29]. IL-1 is not directly mitogenic for

T-lymphocytes, but it induces the production of cytokines such as IL-2, IL-4, IFNγ, and CSF, and the expression of IL-2 receptors, thus functioning as a second signal in T-cell activation [30]. Through enhancing the effects of B-cell factors, such as IL-4, IL-5, and IL-6, it also may influence B-cell growth and differentiation indirectly [31]. Macrophages are activated by IL-1 in an autocrine fashion to synthesize prostaglandin E_2, to produce cytokines, and to increase their cytotoxic activity [23,29]. IL-1 stimulates fibroblasts to proliferate, to produce collagen, and to release prostaglandins and other cytokines [32]. Under the influence of IL-1, endothelial cells release platelet activating factor, endothelial cell procoagulant activity, and plasminogen activator inhibitor, and express higher amounts of intercellular adhesion molecule-1 (ICAM-1) on their surface, which supports adherence of neutrophils, monocytes, and lymphocytes to endothelial cells [33–35]. Moreover, IL-1 induces fever, causes metabolic changes, hypalbuminemia, proteolysis, and increased production of acute-phase proteins, such as fibrinogen, C-reactive protein, and serum amyloid A [36]. Recently, it was observed that IL-1 induces the release of hypothalamic and pituitary gland hormones, including endorphins, corticotropin releasing factor, ACTH, somatostatin, and melanocyte stimulating hormone (MSH) [37,38]. IL-1 also upregulates MSH receptor expression on melanocytes and melanoma cells, as well as melanin production, in the presence of MSH [38]. The observation that MSH blocks the biological activity of IL-1 supports the concept of a self-regulatory feedback mechanism.

Since epidermal cells, in particular keratinocytes, were one of the first cells discovered that did not belong to the macrophage/monocyte lineage that were able to release IL-1 [23], and since IL-1 has been found in significant amounts within the epidermis, it also appeared to be of interest to investigate whether melanocytes and melanoma cells can produce this mediator [39]. Initially a thymocyte and fibroblast proliferation augmenting activity was demonstrated in melanoma-cell-derived supernatants, which according to its biochemical characterization could not be separated from IL-1 [40]. This was further confirmed by neutralizing studies using IL-1α-specific antibodies and by immunoprecipitation. Upon HPLC chromatofocusing, a major peak at pH 5.0, corresponding to IL-1α, and a minor one at pH 7.0, probably due to IL-1β, was observed. These biological data were also confirmed at the molecular level; Northern blot analysis demonstrated the expression of mRNA encoding for IL-1α (Figure 1) [39] and, though in minor amounts, also for IL-1β [41]. Therefore, as with keratinocytes, the major form of IL-1 produced by melanoma cells appears to be IL-1α. It has not yet been determined whether these cells exhibit the capacity to release the specific protease that cleaves the IL-1β precursor into the active 17-kD molecule. There is an obvious heterogeneity within different melanoma cell lines concerning the ability to produce IL-1. The constitutive release in most melanomas is quite low, but can be significantly upregulated by various stimuli such as tumor promotors, lipopolysccharide (LPS), a streptococcus pyogenes preparation (OK432), silica, hydroxyurea, and other cytokines [39,40]. Detection of

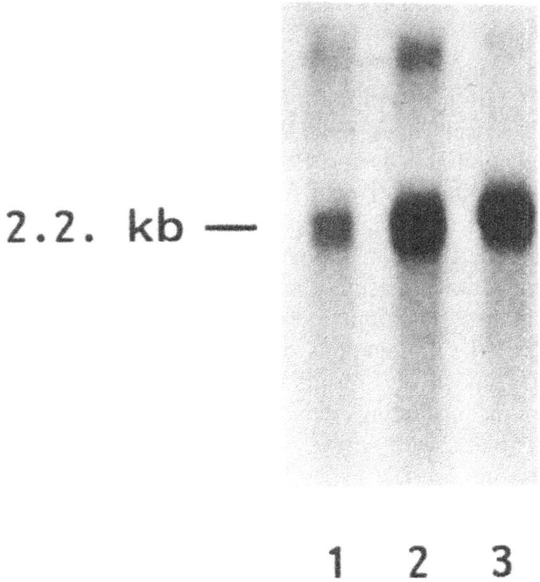

Figure 1. Northern blot analysis of the expression of IL-1α in human melanoma cells. KRFM cells were incubated for 12 hours without stimulus (lane 1) or in the presence of PMA (50 ng/ml, lane 2) and rhIL 1α (5 U/ml, lane 3), respectively. For Northern blot analysis of total cellular RNA (20 μg) a ^{32}P-labeled cDNA probe encoding for IL-1α was used. (Reprinted from J. Natl. Cancer Inst. 81:36–41 (1989) with copyright permission from Editorial Office, R.A. Bloch International Cancer Information Center, Bethesda, MD.)

enhanced expression of IL-1-specific mRNA after cell treatment demonstrates, that these stimuli affect IL-1 production not only at the protein, but also at the gene level (Figure 1) [39].

3.2. Interleukin-6 (IL-6)

IL-6 is a multifunctional cytokine that was discovered independently by various groups and was described according to the respective biological activities under various names, such as B-cell stimulatory factor-2 [42], interferon β2 [9], hybridoma growth factor [43], hepatocyte stimulating factor [44], macrophage granulocyte inducer-2 [45], and 26-kD protein [46]. Macrophages and fibroblasts were originally regarded as the predominant cellular source of this cytokine, however, soon other cells, including endothelial cells, keratinocytes, as well as carcinoma and myeloma cell lines, were demonstrated to exhibit the capacity to release this mediator [47–49]. The constitutive production of IL-6 in general is quite low, but can be significantly upregulated by inflammatory cytokines such as IL-1, TNFα, PDGF, and IFN [50]. In addition, tumor protomors, LPS, different viruses, abnormal nucleic acids, and UV-light are potent inducers of IL-6 synthesis and release [50,51].

IL-6 is an important mediator of B-cell growth and differentiation [52]. It induces the proliferation of murine hybridoma/plasmacytoma cell lines and EBV-transformed B-cell lines [53,54], and it enhances immunoglobulin production in activated B-cells and B-lymphoblastoid cell lines [55]. Moreover, IL-6 may also influence T-cells functioning as a second signal [56] and stimulate indirectly NK cells via inducing the release of IL-2 [57].

IL-6 is also regarded as a mediator of the acute-phase response, since it enhances the production of acute-phase reactants, such as CRP and chymotrypsin, and induces hypalbuminemia [58]. In addition, IL-6 has been identified as one of the endogenous pyrogens, since injection of IL-6 into rabbits and dogs, respectively, results in fever [59]. These observations are also confirmed by recent findings demonstrating significantly enhanced IL-6 serum levels in patients with severe burns [60], septicemia [61], extensive psoriasis [62], after intense UV-exposure [63], and following the injection of endotoxin [64].

The role of IL-6 in the pathogenesis of malignant diseases is still controversial, since several tumors exhibit the capacity to release IL-6 and since some neoplastic cells, such as distinct myeloma cell lines, require IL-6 as an autocrine growth factor [65]. Recent observations also demonstrate that IL-6 stimulates pheochromocytoma cell lines to differentiate into neurite extending cells and to express several protooncogenes at a higher level [66]. On the other hand, IL-6 affects certain fibroblasts and tumor cell lines in an antiproliferative manner [67]. This antiproliferative effect was also demonstrated in breast ductal carcinoma cells; however, it is associated with a disaggregation of cell colonies and an increase in cell motility [68]. How these findings relate to the capacity to metastasize remains to be determined.

Considering these latter observations, it appears to be of interest whether or not IL-6 may have similar effects on melanoma cells and whether or not melanoma cells release IL-6. Recently, two melanoma cell lines were screened for IL-6 production. Using a hybridoma cell growth assay, IL-6 activity was detected in only one cell line after stimulation with PMA [69]. This was also confirmed by Northern blot analysis, which demonstrated no constitutive IL-6 mRNA expression, but significant amounts after treatment with PMA. As with IL-1, there seems to be a heterogeneity within different melanoma cell lines regarding the capacity to produce IL-6. Preliminary observations also indicate that normal human melanocytes release IL-6 after stimulation (unpublished observations).

Previously, it was observed that melanoma cell lines that are similar to keratinocytes release a mediator that activates NK cells and that is distinct from IL-1, IL-2, or IFNγ, and therefore is called epidermal-cell-derived natural killer cell factor (ENKAF) [70,71]. Since both keratinocytes and melanoma cells produce IL-6, and since IL-6 activates NK cells, it appeared to be likely that ENKAF and IL-6 are identical. This was further confirmed by the recent finding that ENKAF activity can be blocked by IL-6 antibodies [71].

3.3. *Interleukin-8 (IL-8)*

Recently, a new group of related human-monocyte-derived mediators that are chemotactic for neutrophilic granulocytes was isolated, purified, sequenced, and cloned by several groups and named neutrophil activating factor (NAF) [72], neutrophil activating peptide (NAP) [73], and monocyte-derived neutrophil chemotactic factor (MDNCF) [74]. Currently, in accordance with the cytokine nomenclature, this mediator has been termed IL-8 [18]. The sequence of IL-8 shows strong homology to previously characterized mediators, such as platelet basic protein [75], β-thromboglobulin [76], platelet factor-4 [77], IFNγ-inducible protein (IP10) [78], v-src inducible protein [79], and melanoma growth stimulatory activity (MGSA) [80].

IL-8 is able to evoke all responses observed in chemotactically activated neutrophils. It induces the release of storage enzymes, produces reactive oxygen metabolites, increases cytosolic free Ca^{2+}, activates the respiratory burst, and induces granule exocytosis [18]. IL-8 acts via specific cell surface receptors, which appear to be distinct from those of C_{5a}, f-Met-Leu-Phe, PAF, and LTB_4 [81], and appears to be very selective, since it does not stimulate phagocytes, platelets, and fibroblasts. However, in addition to its neutrophil-activating capacities, IL-8 was recently shown to function as a chemotattractant for T-lymphocytes and epidermal cells [82,83]. IL-8 is not species specific, and intravenous injection induces granulocytosis and intradermal application results in a massive infiltration by neutrophils and lymphocytes [84].

IL-8 was originally described as a product of monocytes, which release this factor upon appropriate stimulation, including LPS, PMA, Con A, IL-1, TNFα, or IFNγ [72,78]. Recently, however, it was found that fibroblasts, hepatocytes, and endothelial and epithelial cells release IL-8 [73,74,85]. Keratinocytes also appear as a source for this cytokine, since chemotactic peptides obtained from psoriatic scales are identical to IL-8 [85,86].

A protein derived from human melanoma cells that stimulates the growth of melanoma cells was previously isolated and called melanoma growth stimulating activity (MGSA) [87,88]. Recently, MGSA was cloned [80] and turned out to be structurally similar to IL-8 and to exhibit 50% sequence homology with IL-8 [89]. In addition, the human MGSA gene was mapped to chromosome 4, a region that also contains the genes for platelet factor-4, IP-10, and IL-8 [80]. MGSA mRNA was detected in a variety of cell types, including melanoma cells; the level of MGSA mRNA in these cells was strongly enhanced by treatment with MGSA [80]. Therefore, it may function as an autocrine growth factor for melanoma cells. The relation between MGSA and IL-8 recently became more obvious, since it was demonstrated that MGSA is a neutrophil activator and that a minor neutrophil enzyme releasing activity purified from LPS-treated macrophages was due to MGSA [89].

Considering the similarity between MGSA and IL-8, the question arises as to whether melanoma cells can produce IL-8. Recent observations from our laboratory and others indicate that melanoma cells do produce IL-8 which has been demonstrated both at the protein and the mRNA level (124; C. Zachariae, Arhus, personal communication). However, it is not yet clear whether IL-8 similar to MGSA stimulates its own production, as well as melanoma cell proliferation, thus functioning as an autocrine growth factor.

4. Growth regulatory peptides produced by melanoma cells

4.1. Hematopoietic growth factors

Cytokines affecting hematopoiesis were named colony-stimulating factors (CSF) according to their capacity to induce colony formation in soft agar cultures. These factors include interleukin-3 (IL-3), granulocyte-colony stimulating factor (G-CSF), macrophage-colony stimulating factor (M-CSF), and granulocyte/macrophage-colony stimulating factor (GM-CSF) [16,90]. IL-3, also called multi-CSF, and GM-CSF, stimulates the growth of multi-lineage colonies containing erythrocytes, granulocytes, monocytes, and megakaryocytes, whereas G-CSF mainly induces colonies of neutrophils and M-CSF that are primarily monocytes [91].

4.1.1. Interleukin-3. Human IL-3 is a highly glycosylated molecule exhibiting molecular weight heterogeneity between 14 kD and 28 kD. IL-3 and GM-CSF have overlapping and synergistic activities, IL-3, however, is more effective in stimulating more primitive progenitors. In addition, IL-3 is a potent growth factor for colonies containing basophils and mast cells. T-lymphocytes have been regarded as the only cellular source for IL-3. Recently, however, mRNA encoding for murine IL-3 has been detected in murine keratinocyte cell lines, and a mediator stimulating the proliferation of IL-3-dependent cell lines has been observed in supernatants of murine epidermal cells [92,93]. In contrast to the murine system, it was not possible to detect IL-3 mRNA expression in human keratinocytes, supporting the concept that T-cells are the only source for human IL-3. Recently, however, we were able to demonstrate that supernatants derived from the human melanoma cell line KRFM significantly enhanced the proliferation of the IL-3- and GM-CSF-dependent cell line AML193 [94]. This activity could be blocked only partially by the addition of an anti-GM-CSF antibody, while the combination of anti-IL-3 and anti-GM-CSF completely suppressed the melanoma-mediated AML193 cell proliferation. This indicates that KRFM cells, in addition to GM-CSF, produce an IL-3-like mediator. Upon HPLC gel filtration and Western blot analysis, KRFM-derived IL-3 exhibited a molecular weight of approximately 17 kD. Northern blot analysis using a human IL-3 cDNA probe revealed that non stimulated melanoma cells expressed low levels of IL-3 mRNA, which were significantly upregulated by tumor promoters. These findings represent the first observation of a 'non-T-cell' being able to synthesize and release human IL-3.

4.1.2. Granulocyte macrophage colony stimulating factor. Similar to IL-3, GM-CSF exhibits a wide spectrum of biological activities: It supports the proliferation of macrophage, eosinophilic, and neutrophilic colonies and is able to support, in synergy with erythropoietin, the proliferation of erythrocyte and megakaryocyte progenitors. Moreover, GM-CSF enhances the activity of mature granulocytes and monocytes [95]. In contrast to IL-3, the production of GM-CSF is not confined to T-cells, but has been demonstrated in monocytes, fibroblasts, and endothelial cells [15]. Recently, it was shown that keratinocytes may also function as a source for GM-CSF [96]. The release of this factor by keratinocytes may be of major relevance in vivo, since GM-CSF currently has been identified to support the maturation of epidermal Langerhans cells into potent immunostimulatory dendritic cells [97].

Since melanoma-derived supernatants supported the proliferation of the GM-CSF and IL-3-dependent cell line AML193, and since this activity could be partially blocked by anti-GM-CSF antibodies, it was obvious that melanoma cells, in addition to IL-3, also release GM-CSF [98]. This was also confirmed at the molecular level, demonstrating that melanoma cells express mRNA encoding for GM-CSF. Similar to other cytokines, the constitutive production was minimal, but could be enhanced significantly by treating cells with PMA.

4.2. Tumor growth factors

Polypeptide hormones known collectively as growth factors have raised much interest since some of these mediators have been shown to affect the growth of malignant and nonmalignant cells in vitro, suggesting a possible role in the control of neoplastic proliferation [99].

4.2.1. Transforming growth factors (TGF) and epidermal growth factor (EGF). EGF was the first growth factor discovered, when salivary gland extracts injected into newborn mice were found to induce earlier eyelid opening [100]. This 53-amino acid single chain peptide is also involved in the control of gastric acid secretion and enhances normal cell growth and repair processes [101,102]. The search for cancer-specific factors that induce a transformed phenotype in normal cells led to the discovery of TGFα, which is closely related to EGF, but, however, is released in abnormal amounts by some tumor cells. TGFα was first isolated from virus-transformed rat cells and from a human melanoma cell line [103]. Although there is only partial sequence homology, EGF and TGFα bind to the same receptor [104]. TGFα has been reported to be a more potent angiogenic factor than EGF and to be more effective in the induction of osteoclasts [105]. EGF and TGFα are essential for the ability of normal epithelial cell clones to grow. Human keratinocytes express specific high-affinity receptors for EGF, suggesting an important role of EGF and TGFα in the promotion of wound healing, which recently has been confirmed by clinical studies [106,107].

Another peptide in the crude growth factor preparations was isolated that had growth-promoting activity only in the presence of EGF. This factor, called TGFβ, was purified and subsequently shown to either stimulate or inhibit cell proliferation, depending on the experimental conditions [108]. TGFβ does not interact with the EGF receptor and has no relationship with TGFα, except for the fact that both factors were detected in the same supernatant preparations. TGFβ is a homodimer and exhibits a molecular weight of 25 kD. There are three known forms of TGFβ — TGFβ1, TGFβ2, and TGFβ3 — resulting from homodimeric or heterodimeric combinations of subunits [109]. Besides its bimodal effect on cell proliferation, TGFβ blocks adipogenesis, myogenesis, and hematopoiesis; promotes chondrogenesis; and stimulates the expression of fibronectin and collagens in fibroblasts. In addition, TGFβ recently turned out to be a potent immunosuppressor that was blocking the biological activity of IL-1 and IL-3, suggesting a possible role in the downregulation of the immune response [110,111].

TGFα usually is produced by retrovirally transformed cells, by most human tumor cells, and even by some normal cells, e.g., keratinocytes [112,113]. Initially TGFα was isolated and characterized from a human melanoma cell line [103]. It was later demonstrated that melanoma cells also release TGFβ, which was isolated in melanoma cell supernatants by its activity in inducing loose, dispersed colonies in rat kidney fibroblasts [114]. Recently, the production of TGFβ1 by melanoma cells was also detected at the transcriptional level [115]. Since melanoma lines appear to be a source for transforming growth factors, it may be possible that these mediators function in an autocrine or paracrine manner. Accordingly, the transforming activity found in melanoma supernatants characterized by the stimulation of anchorage-independent growth of fibroblasts appears to be due to TGFα, while induction of the anchorage-dependent growth of melanoma cells is due to MGSA [88].

4.2.2. Platelet-derived growth factor (PDGF). PDGF was first isolated from platelets [116]. It is a 30-kD molecule consisting of two peptide chains, termed A and B, which are approximately 60% homologous with one another in terms of their amino acid sequence. The B-chain is encoded by the c-*sis*-protooncogene, the human homologue of the oncogene encoded by the simian sarcoma virus [117]. Most of PDGF purified from human platelets consists of PDGF-AB, and the remainder is principally PDGF-BB, together with small amounts of PDGF-AA [118]. PDGF induces several biological effects on cells by binding to specific cell surface receptors [119,120]. These receptors consist of two subunits, α and β, and each PDGF monomer binds to one receptor subunit; binding studies, however, show that the α subunit can only associate with PDGF-B. Since the detection of PDGF in platelets, it has been observed that both PDGF chains can be produced by many other cells, such as macrophages, endothelial cells, smooth muscle cells, and keratinocytes [120–122]. In addition, many transformed cells, e.g., cells derived from colon carcinomas, hepatomas, and bladder carcinomas, can release either PDGF-AA or PDGF-BB. Some of these cells express PDGF receptors to which PDGF secreted by the same cell can bind, and thus cause tumor expansion in an autocrine manner. Other tumor cells have no receptors but can secrete PDGF, which may affect surrounding connective tissue cells, inducing fibrosis and stroma proliferation. PDGF production can be induced by various stimuli, including cytokines such as IL-1 or TGFβ [118].

Similar to other growth factors, the biological effects of PDGF are pleiotropic [119]. PDGF has been shown to induce the generation of eicosanoides, to modify connective tissue matrix formation, and to be chemotactic for fibroblasts and smooth muscle cells. PDGF is directly mitogenic for cells expressing PDGF receptors such as fibroblasts, vascular smooth muscle cells, glial cells, and chondrocytes. In addition, it enhances indirectly the proliferation of antigen-specific T-cells and MHC class II antigen expression on accessory cells.

Involvement of PDGF in human malignancy is suggested by the finding of expression of the *sis*-oncogene and/or production of PDGF-like activity in a number of human cell lines, including those of neural crest origin [117]. Therefore, various melanoma cell lines were tested for their capacity to produce PDGF. PDGF receptor competing activity was first observed in melanoma-cell-derived supernatants, but not in melanocyte-conditioned medium, suggesting that melanoma cells can produce PDGF [123]. These data were recently confirmed by detecting immunoreactive PDGF using ELISA. In addition, PDGF mRNA was first demonstrated in three melanoma cell lines, one derived from a primary and two from metastases of the same patient. All three cell lines contained a relative abundance of PDGF-A chain transcripts, whereas the primary line expressed B-chain mRNA. As is the case with other cytokines, the production of PDGF appears to be heterogenous, since in several other melanoma cell lines neither PDGF-A nor PDGF-B mRNA was detected [124].

4.2.3. Fibroblast growth factor (FGF). FGF was originally isolated from bovine brain and was described according to its capacity to induce the proliferation of primary and established fibroblasts [125]. FGF activity was found to seperate upon isoelectric focusing with an acidic and a basic isoelectric point. Acidic FGF (aFGF) and basic FGF (bFGF) exhibit 55% amino acid homology [126,127]. A variety of growth factor activities that were previously thought to be unique have been recognized to be due to aFGF or bFGF. Due to their capacity to bind to heparin, they belong to the group of heparin-binding proteins. FGF are not only mitogenic for fibroblasts, but also for endothelial cells, and thus appear to play an important role during angiogenesis [128]. Moreover, FGFs are also chemotactic for endothelial cells and induce the expression of plasminogen activators and collagenases. In addition, FGFs induce the proliferation of chondrocytes, myoblasts, osteoblasts, glial cells, astrocytes, and neuroblasts [129]. Acidic FGFs also induce differentiation and neurite outgrowth of the pheochromocytoma cell line PC12 [130].

It is not clear whether FGFs are involved in malignant transformation, however, they are found to be persistently expressed in tumors that maintain the transformed phenotype. Thus FGFs may function as paracrine or autocrine growth factors and, due to their effect on endothelial cells, maybe involved in tumor angiogenesis. Recently, it was shown that bFGFs inhibited the proliferation of certain tumor cell lines derived from Ewing's sarcoma, angiosarcoma, or osteosarcoma [131]. The same bFGF preparation, however, did not inhibit, or even stimulated, the proliferation of other tumor cells, including rhabdomyosarcoma, epidermal carcinomas, and adrenal or pituitary sarcomas. Thus bFGFs may be considered to be bifunctional regulators of tumor cell growth [131].

Normal human melanocytes, unlike pigment cells derived from metastatic melanomas, do not survive when cultured in routine serum-supplemented media [132]. The search for natural growth factors for melanocytes indicated that mitogenic activity is present in bovine brain and supernatants derived from certain cell lines, including those established from metastatic melanomas and human placenta [132–134]. The factor isolated from the brain has been partially characterized as a protein of approximately 30 kD and a slightly cationic isoelectric point. In view of the maintaining evidence that some oncogenes are homologous to growth factors or growth factor receptors, various of these mediators were tested for their ability to support melanocyte proliferation. Only bFGF in the presence of cAMP turned out to be mitogenic for melanocytes [135]. The mitogenic activity could be blocked by an anti-bFGF antibody. Acidic FGF, however, did not stimulate growth, suggesting that melanocytes bear specific receptors for bFGF [135]. Unlike endothelial cells and fibroblasts, which are stimulated by bFGF and also produce this polypeptide, bFGF was not detectable in melanocytes, either as a gene transcript or as an immunoprecipitable protein [136]. However, melanocytes cultured in the presence of keratinocytes survive for several weeks without the addition of bFGF and cAMP. Furthermore, the melanocyte mitogenic activity detected in keratinocyte-conditioned medium could be blocked by an antibody directed against bFGF. Accordingly, mRNA encoding for bFGF could be demonstrated in keratinocytes. Basic FGF production in keratinocytes is increased after irradiation with UVB light. These data suggest that keratinocyte-derived bFGF is a natural and exogenously inducible growth factor for normal human melanocytes in vivo [137].

In addition, it has been demonstrated that bFGF stimulates the growth of some but not all melanoma cell lines [138]. In contrast to melanocytes, several human melanoma cells produce bFGF, which can support proliferation and thus function as an autocrine growth factor [139].

5. The role of cytokines in the biology of malignant melanoma

There is strong evidence that melanoma cell lines derived from primary and metastatic lesions exhibit the capacity to release several immuno- and growth-regulatory factors in vitro, such as IL-1α, IL-1β, IL-6, IL-3, GM-CSF, IL-8, bFGF, TGFα, TGFβ, and PDGF (Table 1). The production of most of these mediators has been demonstrated at the protein as well as the mRNA level. However, there exists heterogeneity in the capacity to release cytokines within the different melanoma cell lines studied, as no unique secretion pattern by these could be identified. In addition, some melanoma cell cultures turned out to be a potent source for distinct mediators, while others were only weak and some did not produce the respective factor at all. Moreover, there appears to be no general difference in the ability to produce cytokines, whether the cell line is established from a primary or a metastatic lesion. The heterogeneity is also reflected by the inducibility of cytokine release. Stimulation with well-known inducing signals, including tumor promotors, LPS, or cytokines themselves, results in enhanced release by several cell lines that show no or minimal constitutive production. Whether the variable constitutive or inducible productivity is associated with a higher or less aggressive clinical behavior of the original tumors has not yet been pursued.

Cytokines released by neoplastic cells can affect the biological behavior by mediating cell growth in an autocrine or paracrine fashion and by influencing

Table 1. Cytokines released by melanoma cells

	m.w. (kD)	Chromosomal location	Detection in melanoma cells: protein	mRNA	Induction by	Reference
IL-1α			+	+	PMA, LPS, silica	
	17–31	2			hydroxyurea,	39,40,41
IL-1β			+	+	OK432	
IL-6	22–27	7	+	+	PMA	69
IL-8	6–8	4	+	+		124; C. Zachariae personal communication
IL-3	14–28	5	+	+		94
GM-CSF	14–35	5	+	+	PMA	98
TGFα	7	2	+	n.d.		103
TGFβ	25		n.d.	+		115
PDGF	30	7	+	+		123,124
bFGF	18	5	+	+		139

n.d. = not done

defense mechanisms of the host [99]. Basic FGF and MGSA have been demonstrated to be potent growth factors for malignant melanoma in vitro, resulting in an increase of thymidine incorporation and cell proliferation [87,135]. Since both factors are released by melanoma cell lines, they may function as autocrine growth regulators. In addition, bFGF is also secreted by keratinocytes, which through this capacity and through the close proximity to melanocytes may contribute to the growth behavior of early malignant melanocytic lesions [136]. Melanoma cells transplanted into UV-irradiated skin areas exhibit a more rapid growth and an enhanced tendancy to metastasize compared to those cells injected into non-UV-exposed skin [140]. Since keratinocytes have been found to produce higher amounts of bFGF upon UV exposure, bFGF may contribute to the enhanced growth of the melanoma cells transplanted in UV-irradiated skin [136]. As MGSA has recently been sequenced and cloned, specific cDNA probes will be available, and it can be demonstrated by in-situ hybridization whether or not more aggressive melanomas express higher levels of MGSA. There is recent evidence that IL-8 and MGSA are biochemically and biologically related. Therefore, it remains to be tested whether IL-8 may also function as an intrinsic growth factor, similar to MGSA, and whether melanoma cells bear specific receptors for IL-8.

Although melanoma cells can produce TGFα, TGFβ,and PDGF, there is no clear evidence at present as to whether these factors directly influence growth behavior. TGFα, however, is well known to stimulate untransformed fibroblast cell lines to reversibly express a transformed phenotype. Therefore, the correlation between the expression of TGFα and the malignant characteristics of transformed cells, including melanoma cells, in vivo appears interesting from both a biological and a clinical point of view. In addition, growth factors, in particular FGF and PDGF, are chemotactic for endothelial cells and induce the expression of plasminogen activators and collagenases by these cells [119,128]. Therefore, these mediators are likely to be involved in the process of tumor angiogenesis.

The clinical course of malignant melanoma is probably affected by the immune response of the host. Whether particular factors or surface molecules contribute to the fact that some, but not all, lesions are surrounded by a dense lymphocytic infiltrate is at present unknown. Since melanoma cells have been demonstrated to release a variety of immunological mediators, including IL-1 and IL-6, it appears likely that the release of these factors by tumor cells influences the host immune response. Therefore, further studies are necessary to clarify whether there is a correlation between the production of inflammatory mediators by tumor cells and the inflammatory infiltrate. One can speculate that melanomas releasing high levels of IL-1 lead to an early initiation of the immune response by activating lymphocytes and thus inducing the release of other cytokines such as IL-2, TNF, and IL-6. In addition, it recently has been shown that natural and recombinant IL-1β in vitro is cytotoxic to the human melanoma cell line A375 [141]. However, the universality of this finding with regard to other melanoma cell lines and melanoma in vivo remains to be determined.

Recently, several mediators, collectively designated as anticytokines or suppressor factors, have been detected that block the biological activity of distinct cytokines [142,143]. Through their inhibitory capacities, these mediators may play an important role in the downregulation of the immune response and in the induction of immunosuppression. Much information has accumulated on the isolation and characterization of a heterogeneous group of molecules that inhibit the bioactivities of interleukin-1. The altered production of IL-1 and IL-1 inhibitors in tumor-bearing patients and in inflammatory states may contribute to the immune dysfunction associated with these diseases. Among many other cells, keratinocytes, upon UV exposure, have been demonstrated to release a factor that blocks IL-1-induced thymocyte and fibroblast proliferation [144]. Recently, an IL-1 inhibitory activity with similar biochemical characteristics was detected in melanoma cell supernatants [70]. The release of such suppressor factors by melanoma cells may thus impair the immune response of the host and therefore may influence the biological behavior of malignant melanoma.

IL-6 recently has been shown to activate natural killer cells indirectly via the release of IL-2. Since NK cell activity might be involved in the defense against malignant melanoma [145], it needs to be studied whether melanomas that have lost the capacity to release IL-6 exhibit a more aggressive behavior and a poorer prognosis.

Currently, it was demonstrated that the expression of the intercellular adhesion molecule-1 (ICAM-1) on melanoma cells correlates with an increased risk for metastasis [146]. Expression of ICAM-1 may lead to heterotypic adhesion between melanoma cells and LFA-1 expressing leukocytes and thereby may contribute to the dissemination of cells from the primary tumor. However, it remains to be determined whether the increased expression of ICAM-1 on the surface is due to an enhanced intrinsic activity acquired during transformation or whether cytokines released by the melanoma cell itself or by other neighboring cells are responsible for the upregulation of ICAM-1, which can be induced by IFNγ, TNFα, and TNFβ [147].

6. Therapeutic implications for the use of cytokines in malignant melanoma

The observation that cytokines are released by every nucleated cell and that the secretion behavior is usually altered after malignant transformation resulted in the attempt to apply these mediators in cancer therapy [148]. Cytokines can affect tumor growth and behavior in several ways: by exhibiting a direct antiproliferative effect, by activating the host immune response, or by reducing the side effects of conventional cancer therapy. The rationale for the use of the distinct cytokines in clinical trials is mainly based on preclinical in-vitro and in-vivo studies. Interferons and TNFα may have a direct antiproliferative as well as cytostatic effect, whereas IL-2, IL-4, and IL-6 may be used according to their immunomodulatory activity and CSFs because of their capacity to reverse irradiation or chemotherapy-induced myelosuppression [149]. Since there is a great diversity in the growth behavior of malignant melanomas and since the immune response of the host may essentially influence the clinical course, melanoma was one the first tumors included in the biological response modifier (BRM) trials.

In-vitro studies have clearly demonstrated that IFNs are potent inhibitors of melanoma cell growth, as detected both in proliferation and clonogeneic assays [150]. Additionally, IFNs have turned out to be potent immunomodulating agents, since incubation of natural killer (NK) cells — which exhibit spontaneous, i.e., natural, cytotoxicity against a variety of malignant cells, including melanomas — with IFN results in a significant augmentation of NK cell activity [151,152]. Other effector cell functions such as T- and B-cell responses may also be modulated by in-vitro exposure to IFNα and IFNγ [153]. Moreover, IFNγ seems to be a potent signal for monocyte/macrophage activation, resulting in an augmented macrophage cytotoxicity [154]. Another important aspect of immunomodulation by IFN is the enhancing effect on the expression of cell surface molecules on both nonmalignant and malignant target cells [155].

Based on these preclinical findings and promising data from phase II trials [156], recombinant IFNs are now extensively used for the treatment of advanced malignant melanoma and more recently for minimal residual disease (adjuvant therapy) [157,158]. However, objective tumor remission achieved with systemic IFNα therapy in these phase II studies was only in the range of 5–30%, depending mainly on the patient population studied [157,158]. It appears from these investigations that patients with soft tissue metastases and/or pulmonary lesions are those who are likely to repond, whereas bone and/or hepatic metastases are refractory to IFN therapy. Furthermore, the tumor burden is also considered as an important factor, as patients with far advanced disease were found to be weak responders to IFN and other BRM [157,158]. In addition, intralesional injection has also been used to apply IFN in melanoma patients with metastatic disease [159]. Based on these findings, IFNα therapy is now used for the treatment of minimal residual disease, i.e., as adjuant therapy after surgery for melanoma patients with a high risk of relapse [160]. The efficacy of IFNα in combination with IFNγ, IL-2, and TNFα, respectively, is presently being investigated in patients with advanced melanoma [161].

Culture of normal lymphocytes with high concentrations of IL-2 for 3–5 days in the absence of any other stimulus results in the induction of lymphokine-activated killer (LAK) cell activity, which causes a nonspecific lysis of a variety of autologous and allogeneic fresh or cultured tumor cells, including NK-resistant targets [162]. Furthermore, IL-2 injection alone or in combination with LAK cells resulted in the regression of primary and metastatic tumors in a number of murine tumor models [163].

In view of these preclinical in-vitro and in-vivo experiments, recombinant IL-2 has been applied in human malignant melanoma [164]. This approach of combining IL-2 therapy with the infusion of autologous in-vitro activated LAK cells was initially tested in 25 patients with refractory cancer, including melanoma. Eleven of these patients experienced objective tumor remissions [165]. The partial efficacy of this combination therapy was again confirmed by a recent study showing 2 complete, 4 partial, and 1 minor response in 26 evaluable melanoma patients. Furthermore, it was demonstrated in this trial that therapy with a high dose of IL-2 alone also results in a considerable number of tumor remissions [166].

The combined application of IL-2 and IFNα seems to be most promising at present, whereas the combination of IL-2 with IFNγ therapy is just in an early stage of clinical investigation, and therefore no data on efficacy are available [167]. Although the response rates are not at all spectacular, IL-2 and LAK therapy have provided a new impetus for intensive investigations in the field of immunomodulation for the treatment of cancer [167].

At present hematopoietic growth factors appear to be the most efficient BRM in cancer therapy, and their clinical use has expanded dramatically within the last few years. In phase I studies different routes of administration were used to define the optimum biological dose, toxicity and pharmacokinetics of GM-CSF, G-CSF, M-CSF, and IL-3, and it was demonstrated that these recombinant polypeptides can be safely administered over a broad dose range with only minimal side effects [168]. Accordingly, using GM-CSF, G-CSF, M-CSF, and IL-3, new strategies for the treatment of cancer and metastatic melanoma are being developed. Due to the ability of CSF therapy to counteract the complications of chemotherapy, in particular bone-marrow failure and the consequent susceptibility to infection and bleeding, a considerable number of patients, including those with malignant melanoma, seem to be potential candidates for hematopoietic growth factor treatment in combination with standard therapies [169]. Furthermore, these factors may also enable the application of higher and more frequent doses of chemotherapy [169,170]. Moreover, due to the immunomodulating effects of these factors, in-vivo neutrophils and/or monocytes may become more efficient in attacking cancer cells, especially when used in combination with monoclonal antibodies directed against melanoma surface antigens [171]. Other growth factors, such as IL-4, IL-6, and IL-1, are currently being investigated in clinical phase I trials to determine their optimal biological dose and their toxicity [172].

Detection of the optimal dose appears to be an essential requirement for a successful application of BRM, since these mediators can cause severe side effects. This may be due to the fact that cytokines are pleiotropic and exhibit a variety of biological effects, such as vascular leakage, induction of an acute-phase reponse, fever, leukopenia, flulike symptoms, etc. In addition, as demonstrated in vitro, administration of a single cytokine induces the release of other mediators, thus activating the cytokine cascade. Therefore the optimal dosage, i.e., that causing the maximum therapeutic effect with minimal side effects, as well as reasonable but not random combinations of cytokines, need to be determined before cytokine therapy will become an established routine strategy in cancer treatment.

Therefore, the study of melanoma cells as a source for BRM and of their behavior in response to these mediators will contribute to the understanding of the biology of malignant melanoma and will reveal new strategies for treatment [2].

Acknowledgments

This work was supported by 'Fonds zur Förderung Wissenschaftlicher Forschung, grant 7046-MED' and 'Fonds des Bürgermeisters der Bundeshauptstadt Wien, grant 654'. The authors gratefully thank M. Beomer for the excellent secretarial assistance.

References

1. Lee, J.A.H. (1985) The rising incidence of cutaneous malignant melanoma. Am. J. Dermatopath. 7:35–39.
2. Legha, S.S. (1989) Current therapy in malignant melanoma. Semin. Oncol. 16/1:34–44.
3. Boyd, W., ed. (1966) Spontaneous Regression of Cancer. Charles C. Thomas, Springfield, IL.
4. Kradin, R.L., Lazarus, D.S., Dubinett, S.M., Gifford, J., Grove, B., Kurnick, J.T., Pfeffer, F.I., Pinto, C.E., Davidson, E., Callahan, R.J., Strauss, H.W. (1989) Tumor infiltrating lymphocytes and interleukin 2 in treatment of advanced cancer. Lancet 1:577–580.
5. Dumonde, D.C., Wolstencroft, R.A., Panayi, G.S., Mathew, M., Morley, J., Howson, W.T. (1969) Lymphokines: Nonantibody mediators of cellular immunity generated by lymphocyte activation. Nature (London) 224:38–40.
6. Paul, W.E. (1988) Lymphokine nomenclature. Immunol. Today 9:366–367.
7. Schwarz, T., Luger, T.A. (1989) Effect of UV irradiation on epidermal cell cytokine production. J. Photochem. Photobiol. 4:1–13.
8. Dinarello, C.A., Mier, J.W. (1987) Lympokines. N. Engl. J. Med. 317:940–945.
9. Stewart, W.E. II, Blalock, J.E., Burke, D.C., Chaney, C., Durmick, J.K., Falcoff, E., Friedman, R.M., Galasso, G.J., Joklik, W.K., Vilcek, J.T., Younger, J.S., Zoon, K.C. (1980) Interferon nomenclature. Nature (London) 286:110–112.
10. Sehgal, P.B., May, L.T. (1987) Human interferon-β2. J. Interferon Res. 7:521–527.
11. Mestan, J., Digel, W., Mittnacht, S., Hillen, H., Blohm, D., Moller, A., Jacobsen, H., Kirchner, H. (1986) Antiviral effects of recombinant tumor necrosis factor in vitro. Nature (London) 323:816–819.
12. Reis, L.F.L., Le, J., Hirano, T., Kishimoto, T., Vilcek, J. (1988) Anitiviral action of tumor necrosis factor in human fibroblasts is not mediated by B-cell stimulatory factor-2/IFNβ2 and is inhibited by specific antibodies to IFNβ. J. Immunol. 140:1566–1570.
13. Dinarello, C.A. (1984) Interleukin 1 and pathogenesis of the acute-phase response. N. Engl. J. Med. 311:1413–1418.
14. Cerami, A., Beutler, B. (1988) The role of cachectin/TNF in endotoxic shock and cachexia. Immunol. Today 9:28–31.

15. Wong, G.G., Clark, S.K. (1988) Multiple actions of interleukin 6 within a cytokine network. Immunol. Today 9:137–139.
16. Sieff, C.A. (1987) Hematopoietic growth factors. J. Clin. Invest. 79:1549–1557.
17. Mizel, S.B. (1989) The interleukins. FASEB J. 3:2379–2388.
18. Baggiolini, M., Walz, A., Kunkel, S.L. (1989) Neutrophil-activating peptide-1/interleukin 8, a novel cytokine that activates neutrophils. J. Clin. Invest. 84:1045–1049.
19. Luger, T.A., Schwarz, T. (1990) Epidermal cell derived secretory regulins. In: Schuler, G., ed. Epidermal Langerhans Cell. CRC Press, Boca Raton, FL, in press.
20. Roberts, A.B., Frolik, C.A., Anzano, M.A., Sporn, M.B. (1983) Transforming growth factors from neoplastic and non-neoplastic tissues. Fed. Proc. 42:2621–2626.
21. Gery, I., Waksman, B.H. (1972) Potentiation of the T-lymphocyte response to mitogens. II. The cellular source of potentiating mediator(s). J. Exp. Med. 136:143–155.
22. Aarden, L.A., Brunner, T.K., Cerottini, J.C. (1979) Revised nomenclature for antigen-nonspecific T cell proliferation and helper factors. J. Immunol. 134:2928–2929.
23. Oppenheim, J.J., Kovacs, E.J., Matsushima, K., Durum, S.K. (1986) There is more than one interleukin 1. Immunol. Today 7:45–56.
24. Luger, T.A., Stadler, B.M., Katz, S.I., Oppenheim, J.J. (1981) Epidermal cell (keratinocyte) derived thymocyte activating factor (ETAF). J. Immunol. 124:1493–1498.
25. March, C.L., Mosley, B., Larsen, A., Cerretti, D.P., Bradt, G., Price, V., Gillis, S., Henny, C.S., Kronheim, S.R., Grabstein, K., Conlon, P.J., Hopp, T.P., Cosman, D. (1985) Cloning, sequence and expression of two distinct human interleukin 1 complementary DNAs. Nature (London) 315:641–648.
26. Auron, P.E., Webb, A.C., Rosenwasser, L.J., Mucci, S.F., Rich, A., Wolff, S.M., Dinarello, C.A. (1984) Nucleotide sequence of human monocyte interleukin 1 precursor cDNA. Proc. Natl. Acad. Sci. USA 81:7907–7911.
27. Lomedico, P.T., Gubler, U., Hellmann, C.P., Dukovich, M., Giri, J.C., Pan, Y.E., Collier, K., Semionow, R., Chua, A.O., Mizel, S.B. (1984) Cloning and expression of murine interleukin 1 cDNA in *Escherichia coli*. Nature (London) 312:458–462.
28. Kupper, T. (1989) The role of epidermal cytokines. In: Oppenheim, J.J., Shevach, E., eds., The Immunophysiology of Cells and Cytokines. Oxford Press, New York, pp. 285–305.
29. Dinarello, C.A. (1988) Biology of interleukin 1. FASEB J. 2:108–115.
30. Mizel, S.B. (1987) Interleukin 1 and T-cell activation. Immunol. Today 8:330–332.
31. Booth, R.J., Prestidge, R.L., Watson, J.D. (1985) Interleukin 1 and B-cell responsiveness. In: Pick, E., ed., Lymphokines, Vol. 12. Academic Press, New York, pp. 75–86.
32. Schmidt, J.A., Mizel, S.B., Cohen, D., Green, I. (1982) Interleukin 1, a potential regulator of fibroblast proliferation. J. Immunol. 128:2177–2182.
33. Bevilacqua, M.P., Pober, J.S., Majea, G.R., Cotran, R.S., Gimbrone, M.J., Jr. (1984) Interleukin 1 induces biosynthesis and cell surface expression of procoagulant activity on human vascular endothelial cells. J. Exp. Med. 160:618–623.
34. Nachman, R.L., Hajjar, K.A., Silberstein, R.K., Dinarello, C.A., (1986) Interleukin 1 induces endothelial cell synthesis of plasminogen activator inhibitor. J. Exp. Med. 163:1595–1600.
35. Dejana, E., Brevario, F., Erroi, A., Bussolino, F., Mussoni, L., Gramse, M., Pintucci, G., Casali, B., Dinarello, C.A., VanDamme, J., Mantovani, A. (1987) Modulation of endothelial cell function by different molecular species of Interleukin 1. Blood 69:695–699.
36. Kushner, I. (1982) The phenomenon of the acute phase response. Ann. N.Y. Acad. Sci. 389:39–48.
37. Besedovsky, H., Del Rey, A., Sorkin, E., Dinarello, C.A. (1986) Immunoregulatory feedback between interleukin 1 and glucocorticoid hormones. Science 233:652–654.
38. Pawelek, J., Birchall, N., Kupper, T. (1988) Interleukin 1 exhibits dual regulation of the MSH receptor system in cloudman 591 melanoma cells. Clin. Res. 36:682A.
39. Köck, A., Schwarz, T., Urbanski, A., Peng, Z., Vetterlein, M., Micksche, M., Ansel, J.C., Kung, H.F., Luger, T.A. (1989) Expression and release of interleukin 1 by different human melanoma cell lines. J. Natl. Cancer Inst. 81:36–42.

40. Luger, T.A., Köck, A., Wirth, U., Vetterlein, M., Kokoschka, E.M., Micksche, M. (1985) Melanoma cell production of an interleukin 1-like thymocyte-activating factor. In: Bagnara, J., Klaus, S.N., Paul, E., Schartl, M., eds. Pigment Cell, Biological, Molecular and Clinical Aspects of Pigmentation. Tokyo Press, Tokyo, pp. 601–609.
41. Bennicelli, J.L., Elisa, J., Kern, J., Guerry, D.P. IV (1989) Production of interleukin 1 activity by cultured human melanoma cells. Cancer Res. 49:930–935.
42. Hirano, T., Ysukawa, K., Harad, H., Taga, T., Watanabe, Y., Matsuda, T., Kashiwamura, S., Nakajima, K., Koyama, K., Iwamatsu, A., Tsunasawa, S., Sakiyama, F., Matsui, H., Takahara, Y., Taniguchi, T., Kishimoto, T (1986) Complementary DNA for a novel human interleukin (BSF-2) that induces B lymphocytes to produce immunoglobulin. Nature (London) 324:73–75.
43. Braekenhoff, J.P., DeGroot, E.R., Ever, R.F., Pannekoek, H., Aarden, L.A. (1987) Molecular cloning and expression of hybridoma growth factor in *Escherichia coli*. J. Immunol. 139:4116–4121.
44. Baumann, H., Onorato, V., Gauldie, J., Gahreis, G.P. (1987) Distinct sets of acute phase plasma proteins are stimulated by separate human hepatocyte-stimulating factors and monokines in rat hepatoma cells. J. Biol. Chem. 262:9756–98768.
45. Sachs, L., Lotens, J., Shabo, Y. (1989) The molecular regulators of macrophage and granulocyte development: Role of MGI-2/IL 6. Ann. N.Y. Acad. Sci. 557:417–437.
46. Haegman, G., Content, J., Volckaert, G., Derynck, R., Taavernier, J., Fiers, W. (1986) Structural analysis of the sequence encoding for an inducible 26-kD protein in human fibroblasts. Eur. J. Biochem. 159:625–632.
47. Kishimoto, T., Taga, T., Yasukawa, K., Watanabe, Y., Matsuda, T., Nakajima, K., Hirano, T. (1987) Molecular structure and immunological function of human B cell differentiation factor (BSF-2). In: Webb, D.R., Pierce, C.W., Cohen, S., eds. Molecular Basis of Lymphokine Action. Humana Press, Clifton, NJ, pp. 123–136.
48. Santhanam, U., Tatter, S.B., Helfgott, D.C., Ray, A., May, L.T., Sehgal, P.B. (1987) Genetics and function of human 'β2-interferon/B-cell stimulatory factor-2/hepatocyte stimulating factor' (interleukin 6). In: Powanda, M.C., Oppenheim, J.J., Kluger, M.J., Dinarello, C.A., eds. Monokines and Other Non-Lymphocytic Cytokines. Alan R. Liss, New York, pp. 29–34.
49. Kirnbauer, R., Köck, A., Schwarz, T., Urbanski, A., Krutmann, J., Borth, W., Ansel, J.C., Luger, T.A. (1989) Interferon β2, B-cell differentiation factor 2, hybridoma growth factor (interleukin 6) is expressed and released by human epidermal cells and epidermoid carcinoma cell lines. J. Immunol. 142:1922–1928.
50. Ray, A., Tatter, S.B., Santhanam, U., Helfgott, D.C., May, L.T., Sehgal, P.B. (1989) Regulation of expression of interleukin 6: Molecular and clinical studies. Ann. N.Y. Acad. Sci. 557:353–362.
51. Kirnbauer, R., Köck, A., Neuner, P., Förster, E, Krutmann, J., Urbanski, A., Ansel, J.C., Schwarz, T., Luger, T.A. (1990) Regulation of epidermal cell interleukin 6 production by UV light and corticosteroids. J. Invest. Dermatol., in press.
52. Billiau, A. (1987) Interferon β2 as a promoter of growth and differentiation of B cells. Immunol. Today 8:84–87.
53. Tosato, G., Seamon, K.B., Goldman, N.D., Sehgal, P.B., May, L.T., Washington, G.C., Jones, K.D., Pike, S.E. (1988) Monocyte-derived human B-cell growth factor identified as interferon β2 (BSF-2, IL 6). Science 239:502–504.
54. VanDamme, J., Opdenakker, G., Simpson, R.J., Rubira, M.R., Cayphas, S., Vink, A., Billiau, A., VanSnick, J. (1987) Identification of the human 26-kD protein, interferon β2 IFN-β2), as a B cell hybridoma/plasmacytoma growth factor induced by interleukin 1 and tumor necrosis factor. J. Exp. Med. 165:914–919.
55. Muraguchi, A., Hirano, T., Tang, B., Matsuda, T., Horii, Y., Nakajima, K., Kishimoto, T. (1988) The essential role of B cell stimulatory factor 2 (BSF-2/IL 6) for the terminal differentiation of B cells. J. Exp. Med. 167:332–334.
56. Krutmann, J., Kirnbauer, R., Köck, A., Schwarz, T., May, L.T., Sehgal, P.B., Luger,

T.A. (1990) Antibodies directed against CD3 are potent inducers of monocyte IL 6 production. J. Immunol., in press.
57. Luger, T.A., Krutmann, J., Kirnbauer, R., Urbanski, A., Schwarz, T., Klappacher, G., Köck, A., Micksche, M., Malejczyk, J., Schauer, E., May, L.T., Sehgal, P.B. (1989) Interferon β2/interleukin 6 augments the activity of human natural killer cells. J. Immunol. 143:1206–1209.
58. Gauldie, J., Richards, C., Harnish, D., Lansdorp, P., Baumann, H. (1987) Interferon β2/BSF-2 shares identity with monocyte derived hepatocyte stimulating factor (HSF) and regulates the major acute phase protein response in liver cells. Proc. Natl. Acad. Sci. USA 84:7251–7255.
59. LeMay, L.G., Vander, A., Kluger, M. (1989) The role of IL 6 in fever. Cytokine 1:129.
60. Nijsten, M.W.N., DeGroot, E.R., Ten Duis, H.J., Klasen, H.J., Hack, C.E., Aarden, L.A. (1987) Serum levels of interleukin 6 and acute phase responses. Lancet 2:921.
61. Helfgott, D.C., Tatter, S.B., Santhanam, U., Clarick, R.H., Bhardway, N., May, L.T., Sehgal, P.B. (1989) Interferon-β2/interleukin 6 in plasma and body fluids during acute bacterial infection. J. Immunol. 142:948–953.
62. Neuner, P., Kapp, A., Kirnbauer, R., Schwarz, T., Krutmann, J., Luger, T.A. (1989) Monocytes derived from patients with psoriasis synthesize and release increased levels of interleukin 6. J. Invest. Dermatol. 92:490.
63. Urbanski, A., Schwarz, T., Neuner, P., Krutmann, J., Kirnbauer, R., Köck, A., Luger, T.A. (1990) Ultraviolet light induces increased circulating interleukin 6 in humans. J. Invest. Dermatol. 94:808–811.
64. Fong, Y.M., Moldawer, L.L., Marano, M.M., Wei, H., Tatter, S.B., Clarick, R.H., Santhanam, U., Sherris, D., May, L.T., Sehgal, P.B., Lowry, S.F. (1989) Endotoxemia elicits increased circulating β2-interferon/interleukin 6 in man. J. Immunol. 142:2321–2323.
65. Kawano, M., Hirano, T., Matsuda, T., Taga, T., Horii, K., Iwato, K., Assoku, H., Tang, B., Tanabe, O., Tanaka, H., Kuramoto, A., Kishimoto, T. (1988) Autocrine generation and requirement of BSF-2/IL 6 for human multiple myelomas. Nature (London) 332:83–85.
66. Satoh, T., Nakamura, S., Taga, T., Matsuda, T., Hirano, T., Kishimoto, T., Kaziro, Y. (1988) Induction of neuronal differentiation in PC12 cells by B cell stimulatory factor 2/interleukin 6. Mol. Cell. Biol. 8:3546–3549.
67. Revel, M., Zilberstein, A., Ruggieri, R.M., Chen, L., Mory, Y., Rubinstein, M., Michalevicz, R. (1987) Human IFN-beta-2: A cytokine with multiple functions in infections and inflammation. In: Powanda, M.C., Oppenheim, J.J., Kluger, M.J., Dinarello, C.A., eds. Monokines and Other Non-Lymphocytic Cytokines. Alan R. Liss, New York, pp. 21–27.
68. Tamm, I., Cardinale, I., Krueger, J., Murphy, J.S., May, L.T., Sehgal, P.B. (1989) Interleukin 6 decreases cell-cell association and increases motility of ductal breast carcinoma cells. J. Exp. Med. 170:1649–1669.
69. Köck, A., Micksche, M., Vetterlein, M., Schwarz, T., Trautinger, F., Neuner, P., Ansel, J.C., Damm, D., Luger, T.A. (1989) Distinct cytokine mRNA expression by different human melanoma cell lines. J. Invest. Dermatol. 93:559–560.
70. Köck, A., Micksche, M., Vetterlein, M., Luger, T.A. (1987) Human melanoma cells produce immunostimulating as well as immunoinhibiting cytokines. Lymphokine Res. 6:1402.
71. Luger, T.A., Schwarz, T., Krutmann, J., Kirnbauer, R., Neuner, P., Köck, A., Urbanski, A., Borth, W., Schauer E. (1989) Interleukin 6 is produced by epidermal cells and plays an important role in the activation of human T-lymphocytes and natural killer cells. Ann. N.Y. Acad. Sci. 557:405–414.
72. Peveri, P., Walz, A., Dewald, B., Baggiolini, M. (1988) A novel neutrophil-activating factor produced by human mononuclear phagocytes. J. Exp. Med. 167:1547–1559.
73. Schröder, J.M., Christophers, E. (1989) Secretion of novel and homologous neutrophil-activating peptides by LPS-stimulated human endothelial cells. J. Immunol. 142:244–251.
74. Matsushima, K., Morishita, K., Yoshimura, T., Lavu, S., Kobayashi, Y., Lew, W.,

Appella, E., Kung, H.F., Leonard, E.J., Oppenheim, J.J. (1988) Molecular cloning of a human monocyte-derived neutrophil chemotactic factor (MDNCF) and the induction of MDNCF mRNA by interleukin 1 and tumor necrosis factor. J. Exp. Med. 167:1883–1893.
75. Holt, J.C., Harris, M.E., Holt, A.M., Lange, E., Henschen, A., Niewiarowski, S. (1986) Characterization of human platelet basic protein, a precursor form of low-affinity platelet factor 4 and beta-thromboglobulin. Biochemistry 25:1988–1996.
76. Begg, G.S., Pepper, D.S., Chesterman, C.N., Morgan, R.L. (1978) Complete covalent structure of human β-thromboglobulin. Biochemistry 17:1739–1744.
77. Deuel, T.F., Keim, P.S., Farmer, M., Heinrikson, R.L. (1977) Amino acid sequence of human platelet factor 4. Proc. Natl. Acad. Sci. USA 74:2256–2258.
78. Luster, A.D., Unkeless, J.C., Ravetch, J.V. (1985) Gamma-interferon transcriptionally regulates an early-response gene containing homology to platelet proteins. Nature 315: 672–676.
79. Sugano, S., Stoekle, M.Y., Hanafusa, H. (1987) Transformation by rous sarcoma virus induces a novel gene with homology to a mitogenic platelet protein. Cell 49:321–326.
80. Richmond, A., Balentien, E., Thomas, H.G., Flaggs, G., Barton, D.E., Spiess, J., Bordoni, R., Francke, U., Derynck, R. (1988) Molecular characterization and chromosomal mapping of melanoma growth stimulatory activity, a growth factor structurally related to β-thromboglobulin. EMBO J. 7:2025–2033.
81. Samanta, A.K., Oppenheim, J.J., Matsushima, K. (1989) Identification and characterization of specific receptors for monocyte-derived neutrophil chemotactic factor (MDNCF) on human neutrophils. J. Exp. Med. 169:1185–1189.
82. Larsen, C.G., Anderson, A.O., Appella, E., Oppenheim, J.J., Matsushima, K. (1989) The neutrophil-activating protein (NAP-1) is also chemotactic for T-lymphocytes. Science 243:1464–1466.
83. Hein, R., Schröder, J.M., Christophers, E., Krieg, T. (1990) NAP/IL 8, a human monocyte derived peptide is chemotactic for epidermal cells but not for human dermal fibroblasts. Arch. Derm. Res., in press.
84. Van Damme, J., Van Beeumen, J., Opdenakker, G., Billiau, A. (1988) A novel, NH2-terminal sequence-characterized human monokine possessing neutrophil chemotactic, skin-reactive, and granulocytosis-promoting activity. J. Exp. Med. 167:1364–1367.
85. Schröder, J.M., Christophers, E. (1988) Identification of a novel family of highly potent neutrophil chemotactic peptides in psoriatic scales. J. Invest. Dermatol. 91:395.
86. Fincham, N.J., Camp, R.D.R., Gearing, A.J.H., Bird, C.R., Cunningham, F.M. (1988) Neutrophil chemoattractant and IL1-like activity in samples from psoriatic skin lesions. J. Immunol. 140:4294–4299.
87. Richmond, A., Lawson, D.H., Nixon, D.W., Stevens, J.S., Chawla, R.K. (1983) Extraction of a melanoma growth-stimulatory activity from culture medium conditioned by the Hs0294 human melanoma cell line. Cancer Res. 43:2106–2112.
88. Richmond, A., Lawson, D.H., Nixon, D.W., Chawla, R.K. (1986) Characterization of autostimulatory and transforming growth factors from human melanoma cells. Cancer Res. 45:6390–6394.
89. Schröder, J.M., Christophers, E. (1989) Human melanoma growth stimulating activity (MGSA/GRO) is a neutrophil activator. Cytokine 1:152.
90. Groopman, J.E., Molina, J.M., Scadden, D.T. (1989) Hematopoietic growth factors. N. Engl. J. Med. 321:1449–1459.
91. Clark, S.C., Kamen, R. (1987) The human hematopoietic colony stimulating factors. Science 236:1229–1237.
92. Luger, T.A., Wirth, U., Köck, A. (1985) Epidermal cells synthesize a cytokine with interleukin 3-like properties. J. Immunol. 134:915–919.
93. Luger, T.A., Köck, A., Kirnbauer, R., Schwarz, T., Ansel, J.C. (1988) Keratinocyte-derived interleukin 3. Ann. N.Y. Acad. Sci. 548:253–261.
94. Köck, A., Möller, A., Van Lambalgen, R., Urbanski, A., Schwarz, T., Micksche, M., Luger, T.A., (1990) Human melanoma cells synthesize and release interleukin 3. Arch. Dermatol. Res., in press.

macrophage colony stimulating factor stimulates in vitro mature human neutrophil and eosinophil function, surface receptor expression and survival. J. Clin. Invest. 79:1220–1228.
96. Kupper, T.S., Lee, F., Coleman, D., Chodakewitz, J., Flood, P., Horowitz, M. (1988) Keratinocyte derived T-cell growth factor (KTGF) is identical to granulocyte macrophage colony stimulating factor (GM-CSF), J. Invest. Dermatol. 91:185–188.
97. Heufler, C., Koch, F., Schuler, G. (1988) Granulocyte/macrophage colony-stimulating factor and interleukin 1 mediate the maturation of murine epidermal Langerhans cells into potent immunostimulator dendritic cells. J. Exp. Med. 167:700–707.
98. Köck, A., Luger, T.A., Schwarz, T., Kung H.F., Ansel, J. (1988) Human melanoma cells express mRNA for IL 1α, GM-CSF and PDGF. Lymphokine Res. 7:325.
99. Steel, C.M. (1989) Peptide regulatory factors and malignancy. Lancet 2:30–34.
100. Levi-Montalcini, R., Cohen, S. (1960) Effects of the extracts of the mouse submaxillary salivary glands on the sympathetic system of mammals. Ann. N.Y. Acad. Sci. 85:324–341.
101. Savage, C., Inagamai, T., Cohen, S. (1972) The primary structure of epidermal growth factor. J. Biol. Chem. 247:7612–7621.
102. Todaro, G.J. (1988) Oncogenes and growth factors. In: Orfanos, C.E., Stadler, R., Gollnick, H., eds. Dermatology in Five Continents. Springer-Verlag, Berlin, pp. 11–25.
103. Marquardt, H., Todaro, G.J. (1982) Human transforming growth factor. J. Biol. Chem. 257:5220–5225.
104. Waterfield, M.D. (1989) Epidermal growth factor and related molecules. Lancet 1:1243–1246.
105. Sporn, M.B., Roberts, A.B. (1986) Peptide growth factors and inflammation, tissue repair and cancer. J. Clin. Invest. 79:329–332.
106. Lynch, S.E., Colvin, R.B., Antoniades, H.N. (1989) Growth factors in wound healing — single and synergistic effects on partial thickness porcine skin wounds. J. Clin. Invest. 84:640–646.
107. Brown, G.L., Namey, L.B., Griffen, J., Cramer, A.B., Gancey, J.M., Curtsinger, L.J., Holtzin, L., Schultz, G.S., Jurkiewicz, M., Lynch, J.B. (1989) Enhancement of wound healing by topical treatment with epidermal growth factor. N. Engl. J. Med. 321:76–79.
108. Sporn, M.B., Roberts, A.B., Wakefield, L.M., de Crombrugghe, B. (1987) Some recent advances in the chemistry and biology of transforming growth factor-beta. J. Cell. Biol. 105:1039–1045.
109. Massague, J. (1987) The TGF-β family of growth and differentiation factors. Cell 49: 437–438.
110. Wahl, S.M., Hunt, D.A., Wong, H.L., Dougherty, S., McCartney-Francis, N., Wahl, L.M., Ellingsworth, L., Schmidt, J.A., Hall, G., Roberts, A.B., Sporn, M.B. (1988) Transforming growth factor β is a potent immunosuppressive agent that inhibits IL 1 dependent lymphocyte proliferation. J. Immunol. 140:3026–3032.
111. Keller, J., Mantel, C., Sing, G., Ellingsworth, L., Ruscetti, S., Ruscetti, F.W. (1988) Transforming growth factor β1 selectively regulates early murine hematopoietic progenitors and inhibits the growth of IL 3 dependent myeloid leukemia cell lines. J. Exp. Med. 168:737–750.
112. Coffey, R.J., Derynck, R., Wilcox, J.N., Brinman, T.S., Goustin, A.S., Moses, H.L., Pittelkow, M.R. (1987) Production and auto-induction of transforming growth factor-α in human keratinocytes. Nature (London) 328:817–820.
113. Gottlieb, A.B., Chang, G.K., Posnett, D.N., Fanelli, B., Tam, J.P. (1988) Detection of transforming growth factor-α in normal, malignant, and hyperproliferative human keratinocytes. J. Exp. Med. 167:670–675.
114. DeLarco, J.E., Pigott, D.A., Lazarus, J.A. (1985) Ectopic peptides released by a human melanoma cell line that modulate the transformed phenotype. Proc. Natl. Acad. Sci. USA 82:5015–5019.
115. Bodmer, S., Strommer, K., Frei, K., Siepl, C., DeTribolet, N., Heid, I., Fontana, A. (1989) Immunosuppression and transforming growth factor-β in glioblastoma. J. Immunol. 143:3222–3229.
116. Ross, R. (1989) Platelet-derived growth factor. Lancet 2:1179–1182.

117. Heldin, H.C., Westermark., B (1984) Growth factors mechanism of action and relation to oncogenes. Cell 37:9–20.
118. Ross, R., Glomset, J.A., Kariya, B., Harker, L. (1974) A platelet-dependent serum factor that stimulates the proliferation of arterial smooth muscle cells in vitro. Proc. Natl. Acad. Sci. USA 71:1207–1210.
119. Ross, R., Raines, E.W., Bowen-Pope, F. (1986) The biology of platelet-derived growth factor. Cell 46:166–159.
120. Shimokado, K., Raines, E.W., Madtes, D.K., Barrett, T.B., Benditt, E.P., Ross, R. (1985) A significant part of macrophage-derived growth factor consists of at least two forms of PDGF. Cell 43:277–286.
121. DiCorleto, P.E., Bowen-Pope, D.F. (1983) Cultured endothelial cells produce a platelet-derived growth factor-like protein. Proc. Natl. Acad. Sci. USA 80:1919–1923.
122. Damm, D., Shipley, G., Hart, C., Ansel, C. (1989) The expression and modulation of PDGF in normal human keratinocytes. Cytokine 1:74.
123. Westermark, B., Johnsson, A., Paulsson, Y., Betsholtz, C., Heldin, C.H., Herlyn, M., Rodeck, U., Koprowski, H. (1986) Human melanoma cell lines of primary and metastatic origin express the genes encoding the chains of platelet-derived growth factor (PDGF) and produce a PDGF-like growth factor. Proc. Natl. Acad. Sci. USA 83:7197–7200.
124. Schwarz, T., Köck, A., Förster, E., Berger, C., Ansel, J.C., Luger, T.A. (1990) Different melanoma cell lines vary in their cytokine production capacities. J. Invest. Dermatol, in press.
125. Thomas, K.A. (1987) Fibroblast growth factors. FASEB J. 1:4334–440.
126. Jaye, M., Howk, R., Burgess, W., Rigga, G.A., Chiu, I.M., Ravera, M.W., O'Brien, S.J., Modi, W.S., Maciag, T., Drohan, W.N. (1986) Human endothelial cell growth factor: Cloning, nucleotide sequence, and chromosome localization. Science 233:541–545.
127. Abraham, J.A., Whang, J.L., Tumolo, A., Mergia, A., Friedman, J., Gospodarowicz, D., Fiddes, J. (1986) Human basic fibroblast growth factor: Nucleotide sequence and genomic organization. EMBO J. 5:2523–2528.
128. Thomas, K.A., Gimenez-Gallego, G. (1986) Fibroblast growth factor: Broad spectrum mitogens with potent angiogenic activity. Trends Biochem. Sci. 11:81–84.
129. Gensburger, C., Labourdette, G., Sensenbrenner, M. (1987) Brain basic fibroblast growth factor stimulates the proliferation of rat neuronal precursor cells in vitro. FEBS Lett. 217:1–5.
130. Wagner, J.A., D'Amore, P.A. (1986) Neurite outgrowth induced by an endothelial cell mitogen isolated from retina. J. Cell Biol. 103:1363–1367.
131. Schweigerer, L., Neufeld, G., Gospodarowicz, D. (1987) Basic fibroblast growth factor as a growth inhibitor for cultured human tumor cells. J. Clin. Invest. 80:1516–1520.
132. Halaban R., Ghosh, S., Duray, P., Kirkwood, J.M., Lerner, A.B. (1986) Human melanocytes cultured from nevi and melanomas. J. Invest. Dermatol. 87:95–101.
133. Eisinger, E., Marko, O., Ogata, S.I. Old, L.J. (1984) Growth regulation of human melanocytes. Science 229:984–986.
134. Wilkins, L., Gilchrest, B.A., Szabo, G., Weinstein, R., Maciag, T. (1985) The stimulation of normal human melanocyte proliferation in vitro by melanocyte growth factor from bovine brain. J. Cell Physiol. 122:350–361.
135. Halaban, R., Ghosh, S., Baird, A. (1987) bFGF is the putative natural growth factor for human melanocytes. In Vitro Cell Develop. Biol. 23:47–52.
136. Halaban, R., Langdon, R., Birchall N., Cuono, C., Baird, A., Scott, G., Moellmann, G., McGuire, J. (1988) Paracrine stimulation of melanocytes by keratinocytes through basic fibroblast growth factor. Ann. N.Y. Acad. Sci. 548:180–190.
137. Halaban, R., Langdon, R., Birchall, N., Cuono, C., Baird, A., Scott, G., Möllmann, G., McGuire, J. (1988) Basic fibroblast growth factor from human keratinocytes is a natural mitogen for melanocytes. J. Cell Biol. 107:1611–1619.
138. Richmond, A., Lawson, D.H., Nixon, D.W., Stevens, J.S., Chawla, R.K. (1982) In vitro growth promotion in human malignant melanoma cells by fibroblast growth factor. Cancer

Res. 42:3175–3180.
139. Halaban, R., Kwon, B.S., Ghosh, S., Delli Bovi, P., Baird, A. (1988) Basic fibroblast growth factor fused to a signal peptide transforms cells. Nature 331:173–175.
140. Fidler, I.J., Donawho, C., Kripke, M.L. (1990) Direct exposure to UV irradiation is associated with accelerated outgrowth of melanoma cells. In: Riklis E., eds., Proc. Int. Congr. Photobiol, in press.
141. Lachman, L.B., Dinarello, C.A., Llansa, N.D., Fidler, I.J. (1986) Natural and recombinant human interleukin 1β is cytotoxic for human melanoma cells. J. Immunol. 136:3098–3102.
142. Larrick, J.W. (1989) Native interleukin inhibitors. Immunol. Today 10:61–66.
143. Seckinger, P., Isaaz, S., Dayer, J.M. (1988) A human inhibitor of tumor necrosis factor α. J. Exp. Med. 167:1511–1516.
144. Schwarz, T., Urbanska, A., Gschnait, F., Luger, T.A. (1987) UV irradiated epidermal cells produce a specific inhibitor of interleukin 1 activity. J. Immunol. 138:1457–1463.
145. Yanagawa, E., Uchida, A., Kokoschka, E.M., Micksche, M. (1984) Natural cytotoxicity of lymphoctes and monocytes and its augmentation by OK432 in melanoma patients. Cancer Immunol. Immunother 16:131–136.
146. Johnson, J.P., Stade, B.G., Holzmann, B., Schwäble, W., Riethmüller, G. (1989) De novo expression of intercellular-adhesion molecule 1 in melanoma correlates with increased risk of metastasis. Proc. Natl. Acad. Sci. USA 86:641–644.
147. Hogg, N. (1989) The leukocyte integrins. Immunol. Today 10:111–114.
148. Gutterman, J. (1988) Overview of advances in the use of biological proteins in human cancer. Semin. Oncol. 15/5:2–6.
149. Subcommittee report (1983) Biologic response modifier. NCI Monogr. 63.
150. Schiller, J.H., Willson, J.K.V., Bittner, G., Borden, E. (1986) Antiproliferative effects of interferons on human melanoma cells in the human tumor colony forming assay. J. Interferon Res. 6:615–625.
151. Ortaldo, J.R., Petska, S. (1980) Augmentation of human natural killer cell activity with interferon. Scand. J. Immunol. 12:365–369.
152. Edwards, B.S., Merrit, J.A., Futsibrigge, R.C. (1985) Low doses of interferon alpha result in a more effective clinical natural killer cell activation. J. Clin. Invest. 76:1908–1912.
153. Heron, I., Berg, K., Cantell, K. (1976) Regulatory effect of interferon on T-cells in vivo. J. Immunol. 117:637–642.
154. Territs, M., Serma, G., Figlin, F. (1987) Effect of in vivo administration of interferon on human monocyte function. J. Biol. Resp. Mod. 2:450–457.
155. Epstein, L.B. (1981) Interferon as model lymphokine. Fed. Proc. 40:56–61.
156. Krown, S.E., Burk, M.W., Kirkwood, J.M., Kurr, D., Morton, D.L., Oettgen, H.F. (1984) Human leukocyte (alpha) interferon in metastatic malignant melanoma: The American Cancer Society Phase II Trial. Cancer Treat. Rep. 68:723–726.
157. Legha, S.S. (1986) Interferons in the treatment of malignant melanoma: A review of recent trials. Cancer 57:1675–1677.
158. Kirkwood, J.M., Ernstoff, M. (1986) Potential applications of the interferons in oncology: Lessons drawn from studies of human melanoma. Semin. Oncol. 18/3:48–56.
159. Von Wussow, P., Block, B., Hartmann, F., Deicher, H. (1988) Intralesional interferon-alpha therapy in advanced malignant melanoma. Cancer 61:1701–1074.
160. Kokoschka, E.M., Trautinger, F., Knobler, R., Pohl-Markl, H., Micksche, M. (1990) Long-term adjuvant therapy of high risk malignant melanoma with interferon α2b. J. Invest. Dermatol., in press.
161. Rosenberg, S.A., Lotze, M.T., Yang, J.C., Linehan, W.M., Seipp, C., Calabro, S., Karp, S.E., Sherry, R.M., Steinberg, S., White, D.E. (1989) Combination therapy with interleukin 2 and alpha-interferon for the treatment of patients with advanced cancer. J. Clin. Oncol. 7:1863–1874.
162. Grimm, E.A., Mazumder, A., Zhang, H.A., Rosenberg, S.A. (1982) Lymphokine-activated killer cell phenomenon: Lysis of natural killer-resistant fresh solid tumor cells by interleukin 2 activated autologous human peripheral blood lymphocytes. J. Exp. Med.

155:1823–1841.
163. Mule, J.J., Shu, S., Schwarz, S.L., Rosenberg, S.A. (1984) Adaptive immunotherapy of established pulmonary metastases with LAK cells and recombinant IL 2. Science 255: 1487–1489.
164. Lotze, M.T., Frana, L.W., Sharrow, S.O., Robb, R.J., Rosenberg, S.A. (1985) In vivo administration of purified human interleukin 2. I. Half-life and immunologic effects of the Jurkat cell line-derived interleukin 2. J. Immunol. 134:157–166.
165. Rosenberg, S.A., Lotz, M.T., Muul, L.M. (1985) Observations on the systemic administration of autologous lymphokine-activated killer cells and recombinant interleukin 2 to patients with metastatic cancer. N. Engl. J. Med. 313:1485–1492.
166. Rosenberg, S.A., Lotze, M.L., Mule, L.M., Chang, A.E., Avis, F.P., Leitman, S., Linehan, M., Robertson, C.N., Lee, R.E., Rubin, J.T., Seipp, C.A., Simpson, C.G., White, D.E. (1987) A progress report on the treatment of 157 patients with advanced cancer using lymphokine-activated killer cells and interleukin 2 or high-dose interleukin 2 alone. N. Engl. J. Med. 316:889–897.
167. Editorial (1988) Cancer therapy with interleukin 2: Immunologic manipulations can mediate the regression of cancer in humans. J. Clin. Oncol. 6:403–406.
168. Laver, J., Moore, MAS (1989) Clinical use of recombinant human hematopoietic growth factors. J. Natl. Cancer Inst. 81:1370–1382.
169. Steward, W.P., Scarffe, J.H. (1989) Clinical trials with haemopoietic growth factors. In: Progress in Growth Factor Research, Vol. 1, Pergamon Press, pp. 1–12.
170. Brandt, S.J., Peters, W.P., Atwater, S.K., Kurtzberg, J., Borowitz, M.J., Jones, R.B., Shpall, E.J., Bast, R.C., Gilbert, C.J., Oette, D.H. (1988) Effect of recombinant human granulocyte-macrophage colony-stimulating factor on hematopoietic reconstitution after high-dose chemotherapy and autologous bone marrow transplantation. N. Engl. J. Med. 318:869–876.
171. Weisbart, R.H., Gassons, J.C., Golde, D.W. (1989) Colony stimulating factors and host defense. Ann. Intern. Med. 110:297–303.
172. Herrmann, F., Lindemann, A., Mertelsmann, R. (1989) Polypeptides controlling hematopoietic blood cell development and activation. Blut 58:173–179.

4. Phorbol esters and growth regulation in metastatic melanoma cells

Donald L. Coppock, Jeanne B. Tansey, Suzanne Scandalis, and Larry Nathanson

1. Introduction

Normal cells proliferate rapidly under appropriate conditions, yet regulate their growth when the cellular environment indicates. In contrast, the malignantly transformed cell does not fully respond to environmental stimuli signaling growth cessation. Characterizations of most pathways affecting cellular growth were first established in the fibroblast. Recently, the development of culture systems for many different types of cells makes it possible to begin to analyze the regulation of proliferation in other cell types.

About 2–3% of the cells in the epidermis are differentiated melanocytes [1]. In-vitro culture of melanocytes was extremely difficult until a medium containing the tumor-promoting phorbol ester 12-0-tetradecanoyl phorbol-13-acetate (TPA) was developed. This addition enhanced the proliferative capacity of the melanocytes relative to the other cells that were coisolated with them [2]. How the phorbol ester acts to stimulate the growth of the melanocytes is not well understood.

The differences in the requirements for culture of normal melanocytes and transformed melanoma cells are a starting point for many studies seeking to understand the origins of melanoma. Melanoma cells can be cultured in the same growth medium that supports the growth of fibroblasts, with no additional supplements. Indeed, it is possible to grow murine melanoma cells in a very simple serum-free medium with no underfined constituents [3,4]. The loss of a requirement for growth factors commonly occurs in transformed cells. For example, the PG19 melanoma cell line does not require insulin or the insulin-like growth factors in serum-free medium, while hybridization of these cells to fibroblasts leads to activation of this requirement [4]. Halaban et al. have shown that melanomas express the basic fibroblast growth factor (bFGF) gene while normal melanocytes do not [5].

The genetic lesions in melanocytes that lead to uncontrolled growth have not yet been discovered. The search for a melanoma oncogene using transfection of untransformed NIH 3T3 cells resulted in the discovery of the *mel* oncogene in a human tumor cell line [6], but this gene has not been demonstrated to be of general relevance. The activated *ras* oncogene

L. Nathanson (ed.), MELANOMA RESEARCH: GENETICS, GROWTH FACTORS, METASTASES, AND ANTIGENS.

has been found in some melanomas [7–9], but it is not clear whether this is due to genetic instability or represents a late event in the formation of efficiently metastatic cells. In any case, activation of *ras* does not explain the transformation of the normal to the malignant melanocyte [10]. Cytogenetic studies have suggested that loss of tumor suppressor genes may well be an important step in the transition from the normal melanocyte to the malignant melanoma cell [11,12]. A neoplastic phenotype similar to the transformed melanoma cell has been achieved by transferring the gene for the middle T antigen of the polyoma virus into an untransformed melanocyte-like murine cell line [13]. This transformation eliminated the requirement for the addition of phorbol esters in the growth medium. In a similar type of experiment, transfection of the basic fibroblast growth factor cDNA to normal murine melanocytes led to a loss of growth control and the ability to differentiate in vitro, but did not impart the ability to form tumors in vivo [14].

Some agents that are growth promoting for the normal melanocytes inhibit growth in the malignant melanoma cell. This is true for the phorbol ester 12-O-tetradecanoyl-phorbol-13-acetate (TPA) and agents that raise the level of cAMP [15]. TPA, isolated as the active agent for tumor promotion from croton oil [16], has long been known to be growth stimulatory for fibroblasts in culture [17] and to induce hyperplasia when applied to mouse skin [18]. Phorbol esters bind to protein kinase C and have their tumor-promoting effect by mimicking the endogenous activator of the enzyme diacylglycerol [19]. The acute effects of TPA are thought to be mediated through the protein kinase C enzymes (PKC) [20], while the chronic effects may be mediated by a depletion of protein kinase C.

We have begun to analyze how TPA and other phorbol ester analogs slow growth of metastatic melanoma cells and yet are required for active growth of normal melanocytes.

2. Growth effects of phorbol esters and their analogs

To study the effect of TPA on malignant melanoma cells, we have established several cell lines from metastases removed from patients. In Figure 1A we show that TPA inhibits ^{3}H-thymidine incorporation in two cell lines established in our laboratory, the ORL3 and Demel cells, and the HS294T melanoma cell line [21]. A similar effect is seen on cellular proliferation (Figure 1B). The effect is maximal at 24 hours and cells begin to proliferate slowly thereafter. The inhibition of cell growth was strongest on the Demel cell line, so further studies were continued with these.

The Demel line was established from a metastasis to the lymph nodes of a 62-year-old male. It is amelanotic and grows extremely well in MEM supplemented with 10% serum. The doubling time is about 40 hours. The cell line is subtetraploid, with 50–65 chromosomes (median = 55; n = 40). The

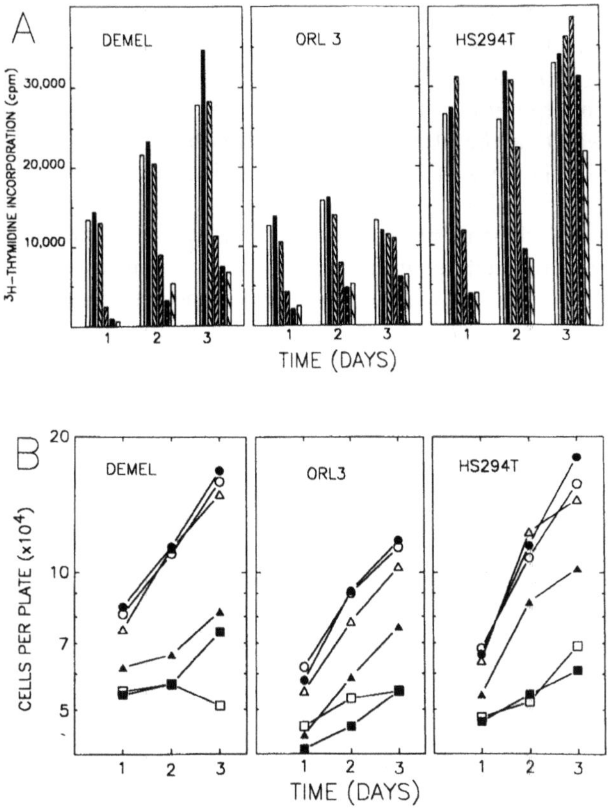

Figure 1. Inhibition of proliferation in metastatic melanoma cells by TPA. The effect of TPA on the growth rate of three melanoma cell lines was measured. A. ^{3}H-thymidine incorporation [key from left to right, no addition, DMSO (0.1%) control; TPA (10^{-9} M); TPA (10^{-8} M); TPA (3×10^{-8} M); TPA (10^{-7} M)]. B. Cellular growth [key: open circle, no addition; solid circle, DMSO control; open triangle, TPA (10^{-9} M); solid triangle, TPA (10^{-8} M); open square, TPA (3×10^{-8} M); solid square, TPA (10^{-7} M]. Methods: Cells: The HS294T cells were obtained from the American Type Culture Collection. The Demel cell line is derived from an amelanotic metastasis to lymph nodes to the breast of a 62-year-old man. ORL3 was established from a melanoma metastatic to lymph nodes of the groin from a 78-year-old female. Growth medium for all the melanomas is minimal essential medium (MEM) supplemented with 2.5% fetal calf serum (Gibco), 7.5% serum Plus (Hazelton), 100 μM penicillin, and 100 μg/ml streptomycin. Thymidine incorporation: Cells were seeded into 24-well plates at 3×10^4 cells/plate and were pulsed at the indicated times with ^{3}H-thymidine (1 μCi/ml) for 30 minutes, the medium aspirated, and 10% trichloroacetic acid added for 15 minutes. TCA treatment was repeated an additional two times, aspirated, the precipitated monolayer was dissolved in 0.2 M NaOH, and an aliquot was counted. Each point is an average of duplicates. Growth curves: Cells were seeded as above, and at the indicated times cells were trypsinized and counted in a Coulter Counter, model ZM.

morphology is cuboidal when grown in growth medium and the cells display increased refractility when cultured in the presence of TPA for 24 hours.

As shown in Figure 1, TPA inhibited both cellular proliferation and ^{3}H-thymidine incorporation at concentrations of 10^{-8} M and greater. One possibility was that the ability of TPA to inhibit cell growth depended on the density of the cells at the time of administration of TPA. As depicted in Figure 2, the ability of TPA to inhibit DNA synthesis over a 24-hour period was not dependent on cellular density, although the amount of DNA synthesis per cell decreased with increasing density.

If the inhibition of growth were induced via the activation and subsequent depletion of protein kinase C, the TPA analogs would be predicted to inhibit to the same degree that they act as tumor promotors. The phorbol ester phorbol 12,13 dibutyrate (PDBu), which is an active tumor-promoting agent for mouse epidermis, was inhibitory for the growth of the Demel cells, while 4α-phorbol (4αP), which is inactive as a tumor-promoting agent, was inactive in the inhibition of growth of the Demel cells. In Figure 3A we show that PDBu is almost as active as TPA, while 4α-phorbol is virtually without activity. The small enhancement of ^{3}H-thymidine incorporation at low concentrations of phorbol esters is frequently observed.

Since the effect of phorbol esters is thought to be mediated through protein kinase C, we measured the effect of two lipid effectors of PKC for the ability to affect the growth of the melanoma cells. sn-1,2-dioctanoylglycerol (DOG) and sn-1-octanoyl-2-acetyl glycerol (OAG) were without effect at concentrations that activate protein kinase C (Figure 3B). The fact that these compounds did not inhibit the growth of the melanoma cells suggests that TPA may be acting through a pathway other than the activation of protein

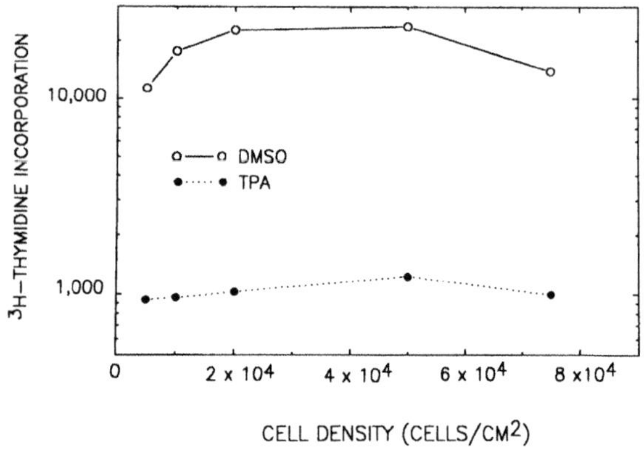

Figure 2. Effect of cell density upon inhibition of growth by TPA. Cells were plated at the indicated densities, ranging from 0.5 × 10^4 cells/cm^2 to 7.5 × 10^4 cells/cm^2. After 1 day either DMSO (0.1%) or TPA (3 × 10^{-8} M) was added. After 24 hours ^{3}H-thymidine was added and incorporation was determined after a 30-minute pulse, as described in the legend to Figure 1.

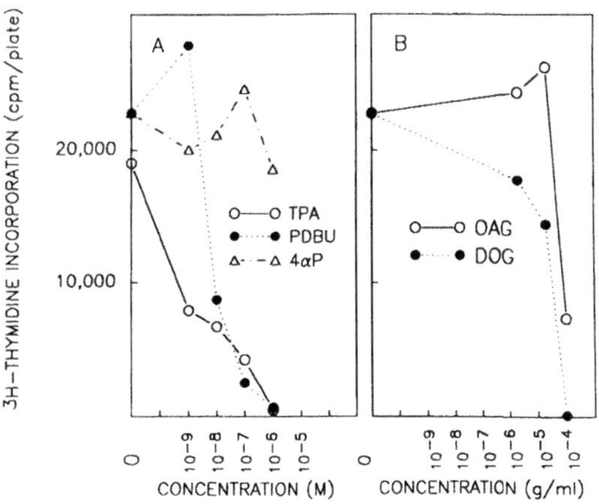

Figure 3. Effect of phorbol esters and diacylglycerol on Demel melanoma cells. (A) TPA, 12, 13-phorbol ester dibutyrate (PDBU) or 4α-phorbol (4αP), or (B) sn-1,2-dioctanoylglycerol (DOG) and sn-1-octanoyl-2-acetyl glycerol (OAG), were added to cultures of Demel cells. Demel melanoma cells were plated at 1 × 10^5 cells per 35-mm culture dish in growth medium. After 1 day additions, as described above, were added. After a 24-hour incubation with the drugs, ^{3}H-thymidine incorporation was determined, as described in the legend to Figure 1.

kinase C. The inhibition at the highest doses was clearly due to generalized toxicity.

Because melanocytes were stimulated rather than inhibited by TPA, it was of interest to examine how TPA analogs affected the melanocytes. We have established cultures of melanocytes and good long-term growth is seen in the presence of TPA without the addition of extracts from other cells (see legend for Figure 8). To test how TPA analogs affected melanocyte growth, they were cultured in medium without TPA for 4 days, including two medium changes, and then medium with various additives was added back to these cell and cellular proliferation was followed. As for the melanoma cells, only PDBU was effective in mimicking the effect of TPA. The diacylglycerols DOG and OAG were ineffective and at the highest doses were clearly cytotoxic. Again, this suggests that cells of the melanocytic lineage are affected by TPA and other phorbol esters through a pathway other than stimulation of PKC.

3. TPA and cell cycle

If phorbol esters inhibited the growth of melanoma cells by acting on a small number of intracellular targets, one would expect the growth arrest to be cell-cycle specific. To test this possibility, we treated the cells with various concentrations of TPA for 24 hours and analyzed them with two-dimensional flow microfluorimetry, as shown in Figure 4. As demonstrated in panel 4A,

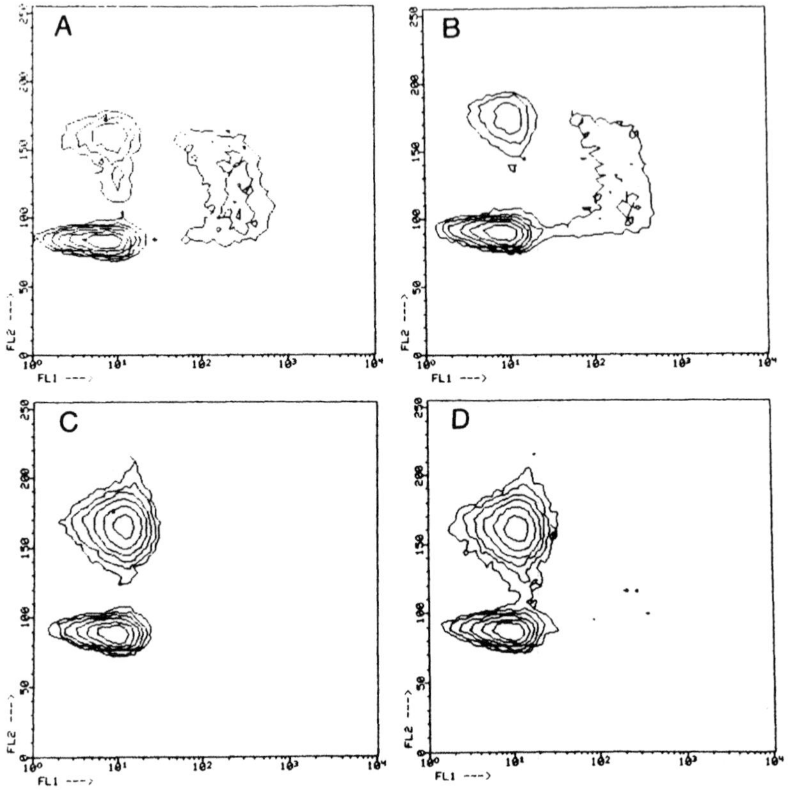

Figure 4. Flow microfluorimetry of Demel melanoma cells treated with TPA. To determine the part of the cell cycle that the melanoma cells arrested in, cells were treated with (A) DMSO (0.1%), (B) TPA (10^{-9} M), (C) TPA (10^{-8} M), and (D) TPA (10^{-7} M) for 24 hours. The FL1 channel shows the amount of green fluorescence (representing the rate of DNA synthesis) and the FL2 channel shows the amount of red fluorescence (representing the amount of DNA per cell). Methods: Cells were pulsed for 30 minutes with 10 μM bromodeoxyuridine (BUdR) at 37°C in a 5% CO_2 atmosphere. At this time the cells were harvested and prepared for flow microfluorimetry by a modification of the thermal denaturation method (as described by Becton Dickenson). Cells were harvested with trypsin, washed, and resuspended in phosphate buffered saline (PBS). Cells were fixed in 70% ethanol (−20°C) and held on ice for 30 minutes. Cells were then treated with 0.25% paraformaldehyde for 30 minutes at room temperature and washed with PBS. They were then treated with RNase, pelleted, and resuspended in 0.1 M HCl with 0.5% Triton X-100. Cells were pelleted and resuspended in H_2O, and the tube was placed in an H_2O bath for 10 min at 100°C. The tube was rapidly cooled and then centrifuged, and the cells were resuspended in 50:50, PBS:2 × SSC (1 × SSC = 0.18 M NaCl, 0.03 M sodium citrate), 0.5% Tween-20, and 1% BSA. Anti-BUdR FITC (B-D monoclonals) was added and incubated for 30 minutes at room temperature, and the cells were washed and stained with propidium iodide. Analysis was performed using a FACSCAN flow cytometer (Becton Dickenson). For each experiment 50,000 cells were counted and contours were drawn using C30 or Lysys software (Becton-Dickenson).

approximately 20% of the cells treated with DMSO were in S phase, 15% in G_2/M, and the rest in G_1. Cells not treated with DMSO are indistinguishable from those in panel A. In panels B, C, and D we see that increasing doses of TPA caused a larger percentage of the cells to accumulate in G_1, a large decrease in the number of cells in S phase, and an increase in the number of cells in G_2.

To test if there were a slow growing subpopulation in this cell line, the cells were labeled for 48 hours with BUdR and then subjected to two-dimensional flow microfluorimetry analysis. As shown in Figure 5A, almost all cells (92%) synthesized DNA (as shown by the incorporation of BUdR) during this period. This is expected, since the doubling time (= average cell cycle length) is about 40 hours. This shows that almost all cells in the population are cycling. To examine the cell cycle arrest in a different way, we asked what happened to cells in S phase after TPA had been added. We added TPA to cultures of Demel cells and after 4 hours labeled them with BUdR for 30 minutes. This labels the population of cells that are in S phase during the 30-minute pulse. The BUdR was washed out and medium containing TPA was restored. After an additional 20 hours, the cells were harvested and analyzed. As shown in Figure 5B, most of the labeled cells were found with G_1 or G_2 DNA content and almost none were found in S phase. This showed that in the

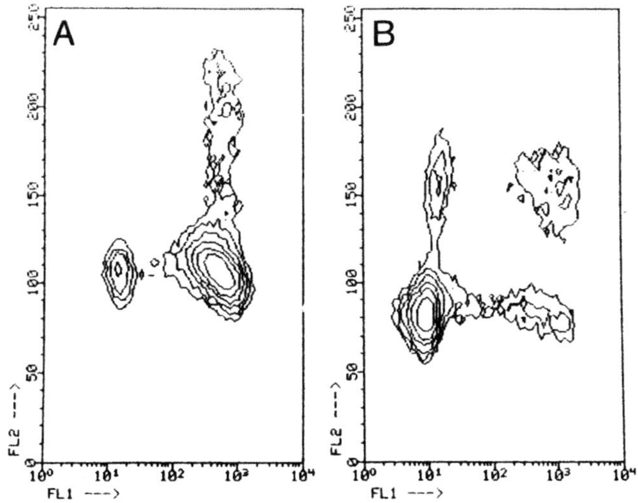

Figure 5. Analysis of effect of TPA on proliferation of Demel cells. A. To determine if there was a population of cells that did not proliferate, cells were labeled for 48 hours with BUdR and then processed for flow microfluorimetry, as described in the legend to Figure 4. B. To determine if TPA blocked cells in S phase, 1×10^6 cells were plated per 100-mm dish and the next day TPA (3×10^{-8} M) was added. After 4 hours BUdR was added for a 30-minute pulse, the plates were rinsed, and medium without BUdR, supplemented with TPA, was added back. The plates were incubated for an additional 20 hours and then analyzed for two-dimensional flow microfluorimetry, as described in the legend to Figure 4.

presence of TPA, cells completed S phase and their growth was arrested in either G_1 or G_2.

4. Kinetics of inhibitory activity of phorbol esters

The inhibition of cell proliferation was determined 24 hours after the TPA was added. By this time it is known that the amount of protein kinase C activity is largely depleted [20]. However, the kinetics of the inhibition of growth of the Demel cells demonstrated that TPA began to act within 1 hour of the time of addition of TPA. As shown in Figure 6, the rate of DNA synthesis began to drop soon after the drug was applied. In contrast, in the presence of staurosporine, which is a potent inhibitor of protein kinase C [22], the Demel cells showed very different kinetics. We chose a dose of staurosporine (3×10^{-9} M) that inhibited DNA synthesis by more than 90% after 24 hours without obvious cytotoxicity. As shown in Figure 6, staurosporine had little or no effect on the rate of DNA synthesis for more than 6 hours, while by 6 hours TPA had inhibited DNA synthesis by more

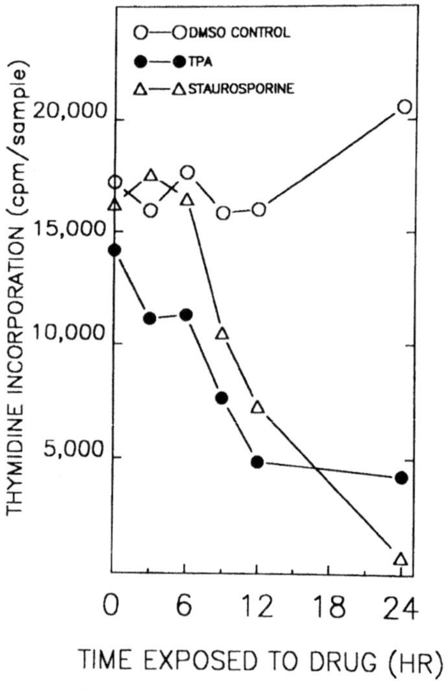

Figure 6. Kinetics of inhibition of DNA synthesis in Demel cells. Cells were plated at 1×10^5 cells/35-mm culture dish. After 18 hours DMSO (0.1%), TPA (3×10^{-8} M), or staurosporine (3×10^{-9} M) were added. ^{3}H-thymidine (1 μCi/ml) was added for 1 hour, beginning at the time indicated, and the plates were processed, as described in the legend to Figure 1.

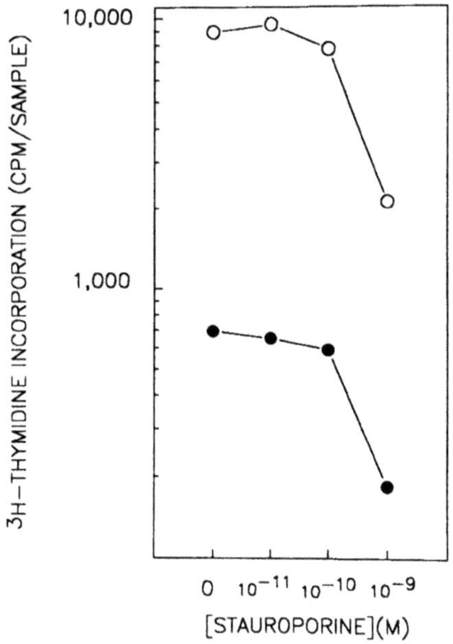

Figure 7. Additivity of staurosporine and TPA. Cells were plated at 2×10^4 cells per well in a 24-well plate. After 24 hours DMSO (open circles) or TPA (3×10^{-8} M, filled circles) and staurosporine at the indicated concentrations were added. After 24 hours ^{3}H-thymidine (1 μCi/ml) was added for 30 minutes, and the plates were processed, as described in the legend to Figure 1.

than 25%. After this time, staurosporine was highly effective in inhibiting the incorporation of ^{3}H-thymidine.

If staurosporine and TPA were inhibiting the growth of the melanoma cells by acting on the same pathway, we would expect that their effects would be subadditive at higher concentrations. However, as shown in Figure 7, TPA and staurosporine are additive in their effects on the melanoma cells. This suggests that TPA is probably not acting solely through those protein kinases inhibited by staurosporine.

5. Is TPA acting by substituting for a growth factor?

Protein kinase C has been implicated in the growth stimulatory pathways for many cell types. Cells with high levels of transfected PKC are extremely responsive to certain growth factors and can be transformed easily [23,24]. Halaban et al. demonstrated that basic fibroblast growth factor (bFGF) is a mitogen for melanocytes that is found in keratinocytes and that it can substitute for TPA in short-term growth assays [25,26]. If TPA and bFGF were acting via the same pathway in Demel cells, we would expect bFGF to be

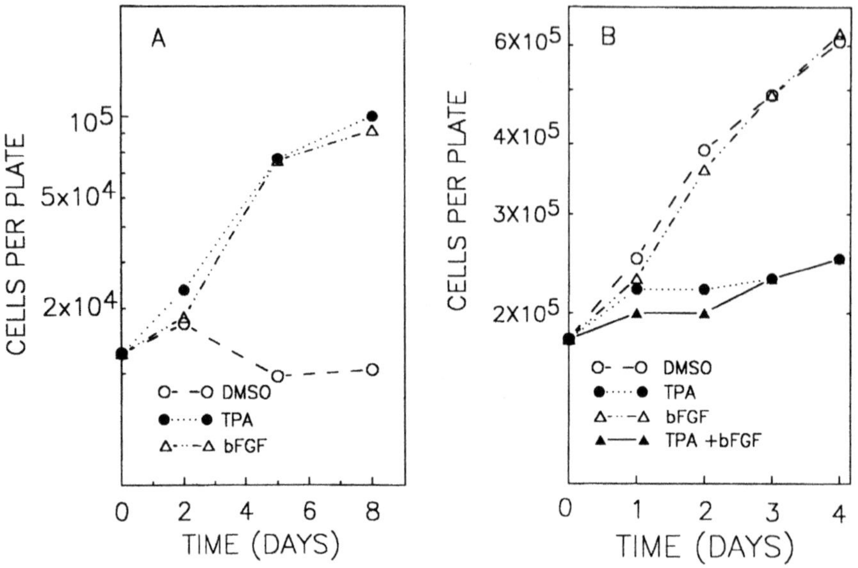

Figure 8. Effect of bFGF on melanocytes and melanoma cells: A. Melanocytes were plated in melanocyte growth medium. After 1 day growth medium was removed and medium without TPA was added. On day 3 fresh medium without TPA was added again. On day 5 medium without TPA supplemented with DMSO, bFGF (1 ng/ml), or TPA (5×10^{-8} M) was added and cell growth was monitored for the following 8 days. B. Demel melanoma cells were plated at 1.8×10^5 cells per 35-mm tissue culture plate and after 24 hours DMSO, TPA (3×10^{-8} M), bFGF (1 ng/ml), or bFGF and TPA were added. Cells were harvested and counted for 4 days following the addition of the supplements. Methods: Cell numbers were determined as described in the legend to Figure 1. The melanocyte cultures were established from human foreskins, as described by Halaban et al. [15,43]. They were cultured in F10 medium (Gibco) supplemented with 5% fetal calf serum (Gibco), 5% serum plus (Hazelton), 0.1 mM isobutyl methyl xanthine (IBMX), 1 nM cholera toxin (List Bilchemicals), 100 μM penicillin, and 100 μg/ml streptomycin in a 37°C incubator with 5% CO_2. Cultures were expanded and then frozen at passages 4–6 and used for experiments in passages 6–20.

inhibitory for growth. In Figure 8A, TPA or bFGF added to melanocytes that had been cultured without TPA for 4 days (with two medium changes) were essentially equivalent for melanocyte growth, but at least one was required. In contrast, bFGF had no effect on the growht of the Demel cells or on the ability of TPA to inhibit their growth (Figure 8B). This suggests that the pathways stimulated by bFGF cannot be identical to those stimulated by TPA.

6. Effect on gene transcription

One possibility is that TPA, which is known to alter the transcription of many genes [27], might be altering the expression of specific isozymes of protein

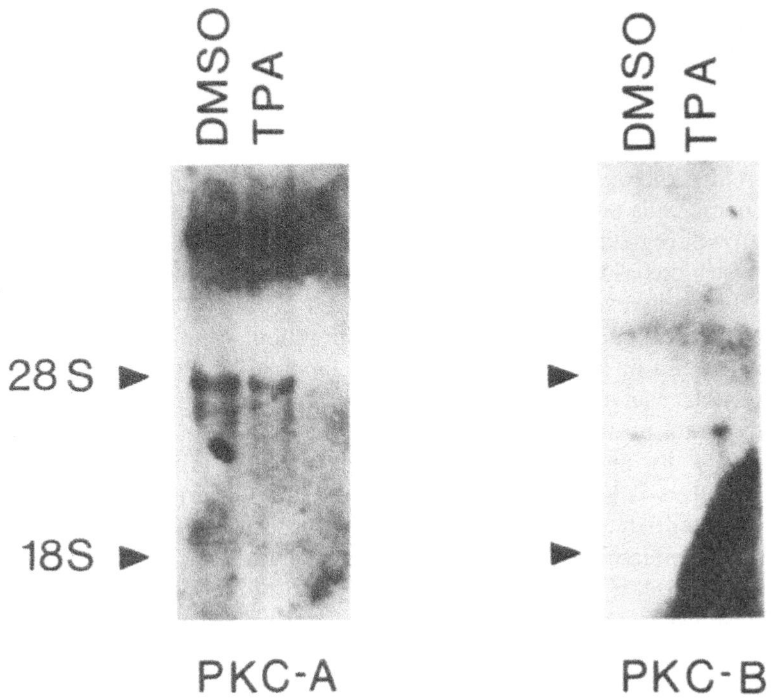

Figure 9. Northern blots of PKCα and PKCβ mRNA in Demel cells. Demel cells were plated in complete medium and after 24 hours DMSO (0.1%) or TPA (3×10^{-8} M) was added. After 24 hours cells were harvested, and Northern blots were prepared and probed with probes to PKCα, PKCβ, and PKCγ [28]. No signal was obtained using the probe to PKCγ. Methods: Northern blots: RNA was prepared by the method of Chirgwin et al. [44], and Northern analysis was performed as previously described [45] using probes to PKCα, PKCβ, and PKCγ [28]. Positions of the 18S and 28S ribosomal RNAs were visualized by UV shadowing.

kinase C. To examine this possibility, we prepared Northern blots of RNA from Demel cells treated with DMSO or TPA and hybridized them to the probes for protein kinase C α (PKC 3), protein kinase C β (PKC 2) and protein kinase C γ (PKC 1) [28]. Signals were detected for PKC α and PKC β; however, TPA treatment induced no change (Figure 9). PKC γ mRNA was not detected under either condition.

7. Discussion

Cellular growth and differentiation in normal vertebrate cells is regulated by interaction with the external cellular environment, i.e., growth factors, extracellular matrix, and cell-to-cell contact. Transformed cells lose this dependence, regulation of growth and differentiation is disturbed, and frequently control completely breaks down. The normal melanocyte is in intimate contact with other cells in the epidermis, e.g., keratinocytes and fibroblasts, both of which produce growth factors that are not produced by the melanocyte [25]. The melanocytes are only a small percentage of the cells in the epidermis, and their growth is precisely regulated. bFGF inhibits differentiation of the melanocytes and is mitogenic [29]. The metastatic melanoma cells are capable of growing outside the epidermis and much of the growth regulation has been lost.

Suggestions as to which growth regulatory mechanisms have been altered have been discovered when these two cell types were cultured. Normal melanocytes require TPA for active proliferation, whether in medium containing serum or in a completely defined medium [2,30]. Although it is not entirely clear as to how TPA is acting in promoting growth, bFGF appears to be able to substitute for TPA in short-term growth assays [25] (Figure 8A). However, the morphology of human melanocytes grown with TPA and bFGF differs [29, our observations]. In addition, murine melanocytes are less differentiated when cultured with a transfected bFGF cDNA [14]. Growth stimulation by bFGF does not appear to require the activation of protein kinase C in murine fibroblasts [31] or CHO cells [32], although both pathways stimulated by both TPA and bFGF may impinge on the same intracellular targets.

Melanoma cells have not been difficult to culture and the success rate is as high as $> 80\%$ [33]. Melanoma cells have relatively simple growth requirements, and they grow well in standard tissue-culture media supplemented with only serum. In contrast to melanocytes, TPA is a growth inhibitor for many melanoma cell lines [15]. This suggests that there has been an overall disturbance in the pathways that regulate growth and differentiation in melanoma cells. TPA apparently acts as an inducer of a more differentiated phenotype, which in turn leads to slowing or cessation of cellular proliferation in several transformed cell types, besides melanoma, including the HL-60 promyelocytic leukemia line [34], human neuroblastoma [35], Daudi Burkitt lymphoma cells [36], and A549 human lung carcinoma cells [37]. The fact that TPA and tumor-promoting phorbol esters cause growth inhibition in several transformed lines derived from distinct developmental lineages suggests that the alteration of this pathway is of fundamental importance for cellular transformation in general.

7.1. Mechanism of action of TPA

How is TPA acting in melanoma cells? It is well known that the TPA receptor in cells is the family of protein kinase C isozymes. These protein kinases are activated by Ca^{2+}, phospholipids, and diacylglycerol, and are thought to mediate the responses of many receptor-activated effects. The enzymes are found in the cytosol and membrane fractions. Within minutes of binding to diacylglycerol or TPA, PKC relocates to the plasma membrane from the cytoplasm and then is proteolytically cleaved into a TPA binding moiety and a protein kinase moiety, referred to as protein kinase M [19]. A 24-hour exposure of many cell types to TPA (10^{-6} M) inactivates almost all PKC activity.

7.1.1. Cell cycle effects of TPA. Our central observation was that application of TPA caused inhibition of growth by preventing cells in G1 from entering S phase and by causing a secondary block that prevented G2/M cells from entering G1. Flow cytometry of a cycling cell population showed that approximately 60–65% of the cells were in G1 and the rest were in S/G2/M (see Figure 4). Our data demonstrated that cells that are in S phase when TPA is applied complete it and then continue through the cell cycle, arresting at G2/M or G1. The observation that TPA caused cell-cycle arrest at two distinct points in the cell cycle raises the question as to whether this is the sum of two distinct activities mediated by TPA or an action that is mediated through a single effector of TPA. Because of the dual nature of the response to TPA, by stimulation and depletion of protein kinase C activity it is possible that a complex range of cellular effects will be seen.

A time course of the addition of TPA to the Demel melanoma cells showed that DNA synthesis began to be inhibited by 1 hour after TPA was administered. In contrast staurosporine, a potent inhibitor of protein kinase C, was ineffective for 6 hours in blocking ^{3}H-thymidine incorporation. This suggests that the initial effect seen might be mediated by the acute effect of TPA, i.e., the activation of protein kinase C, and that the later effects may be mediated by the depletion of PKC that is caused by chronic administration of TPA. It is interesting to note, however, that the effects of PKC and staurosporine are additive across a large dose range. If both drugs acted through the depletion or inactivation of PKC activity, then one would expect their effects to be subadditive at higher doses. In contrast, staurosporine antagonizes the effect of TPA in the induction of ornithine decarboxylase mRNA in mouse epidermis [38]. One possibility that must be considered is that although staurosporine is one of the most specific inhibitors of protein kinase C, it is inhibitory for several other protein kinases and that the additive effects seen are due to a loss of protein kinase C as well as to inhibition of other kinases required for growth. A comparison with the TPA-induced differentiation of HL-60 cells is informative. HL-60 cells differentiate into macrophagelike cells when exposed to TPA concentrations greater than 10^{-9} M. These cells express differentiation-specific antigens but do not proliferate in response to TPA. Dose response curves of HL-60 cells exposed to various concentrations of TPA demonstrate that extremely low concentrations not only fail to activate the differentiation of these cells, but also stimulate a low amount of DNA synthesis in these cells. We have observed a similar phenomenon with low concentrations of phorbol esters (see Figure 3). One possibility is that different isozymes of PKC are activated or proteolytically cleaved at different concentrations of PKC. Huang et al. [39] showed that

PKC III (from the PKCα gene) was degraded more slowly, both in vitro and in vivo, than PKC II (from the PKCβ gene) when exposed to various PKC activators. However, Nishizuka and coworkers [20] demonstrated that these two isoforms were activated differently depending on the presence of diacylglycerol. One possibility that must be explored is whether different isozymes of PKC are responsible for different activities of TPA. The Demel cells contained mRNA for PKCα and PKCβ, but PKCγ mRNA was not detected. This is consistent with the pattern observed in other tissues [20].

Another approach to understanding how TPA acts to induce growth inhibition is to use TPA analogs. TPA is an extremely potent tumor promotor, however, several other phorbol derivatives have different capacities. We tested PDBU, which is also a strong tumor promotor, and 4α phorbol, which has little or no tumor-promoting activity. These two compounds inhibited melanoma cell growth according to their strength as tumor promotors, which also corresponds with their efficiency in causing activation and the eventual loss of protein kinase C activity. In contrast, two diacylglycerols, dioctanoyl and 1-acetyl-2-octanoyl glycerol, were ineffective in growth inhibition of the melanoma cells, except when they were obviously cytotoxic. This appears to be similar to the induction of differentiation of HL-60 cells by activators of PKC. Here the diacylglycerols were shown to induce the phosphorylation of cellular proteins, but failed to cause differentiation and cell-cycle arrest of the HL-60 cells [40]. A similar phenomenon was observed with the A549 lung carcinoma cells [41]. In each of these cases, in transformed cell lines from different developmental lineages, TPA and tumor-promoting phorbol esters are growth inhibitory, but the diacylglycerols failed to inhibit growth unless a cytotoxic level was reached. This suggests that growth inhibition may not be mediated by a mechanism that includes activation of protein kinase C or it may be possible that the inhibition is mediated by only one isozyme of PKC. On the other hand, it may be that complete depletion of PKC following activation is required. The half-life of diacylglycerol is much shorter than TPA, because it is lost from the cell by phosphorylation to form phosphatidic acid.

8. Future directions

To understand the loss of growth control in transformed melanoma cells, the reversal in roles of FGF and TPA in cellular proliferation must be analyzed. An understanding of how gene expression is regulated will be an integral part of this process. TPA induces many of its acute effects by changes in gene expression [27], presumably mediated by phosphorylation of cellular proteins by the isozymes of PKC. Several genes have been found to have a TPA-responsive element in the 5′ controlling region [42]. This site is occupied by the DNA-binding protein complex AP-1 when the cells are stimulated by TPA, certain growth factors, and serum. A depletion of PKC would certainly alter the expression of these genes.

Although both TPA and bFGF are growth stimulatory for normal human melanocytes, they clearly have opposite effects on the differentiation of these cells. The way in which stimulation of gene expression differs in response to TPA and bFGF in these cells will certainly play a major role in determining the phenotypic changes found in the transformed melanoma cells. Since the dysplastic nevus is a premalignant lesion thought to be the precursor of malignant melanoma in about 20% of the cases, it is an important intermediary in the melanocytic lineage. It will be important to know if changes in gene expression induced by TPA are the same in melanocytes, dysplastic nevi, and malignant melanoma cells.

References

1. Frenk, E., Schellhorn, J.P. (1969) Zur morphologie der epidermalen melanineinheit. Dermatologica 139:271–277.
2. Eisinger, M., Marko, O. (1982) Selective proliferation of normal human melanocytes in vitro in the presence of phorbol ester and cholera toxin. Proc. Natl. Acad. Sci. USA 79:2018–2022.
3. Bottenstein, J., Hayashi, I., Hutchings, S., Masui, H., Mather, J., McClure, D., Ohasa, S., Rizzino, A., Sato, G., Serrero, G., Wolfe, R., Wu, R. (1979) The growth of cells in serum-free hormone-supplemented media. Methods Enzymol. 58:94–109.
4. Coppock, D.L., Straus, D.S. (1982) Growth response to insulin and multiplication stimulating activity in mouse melanoma cells and mouse embryo fibroblasts x melanoma hybrids. In: Growth of Cells in Hormonally Defined Media, Cold Spring Harbor Press, Cold Spring Harbor, N.Y., pp. 921–928.
5. Halaban, R., Kwon, B.S., Ghosh, S., Delli Bovi, P., Baird, A. (1988) bFGF as an autocrine growth factor for human melanomas. Oncogene Res 3:177–186.
6. Padua, R.A., Barrass, N., Currie, G.A. (1984) A novel transforming gene in a human malignant melanoma cell line. Nature 311:671–673.
7. Gerhard, D.S., Dracopoli, N.C., Bale, S.J., Houghton, A.N., Watkins, P., Payne, C.E., Greene, M.H., Housman, D.E. (1987) Evidence against Ha-*ras*-1 involvement in sporadic and familial melanoma. Nature 325:73–75.
8. Albino, A.P., Le Strange, R., Oliff, A.I., Furth, M.E., Old, L.J. (1984) Transforming ras genes from human melanoma: A manifestation of tumour heterogeneity?. Nature 308:69–72.
9. Albino, A.P., Nanus, D.M., Mentle, I.R., Cordon-Cardo, C., McNutt, N.S., Bressler, J., Andreeff, M. (1989) Analysis of *ras* oncogenes in malignant melanoma and precursor lesions: Correlation of point mutations with differentiation phenotype. Oncogene 4:1363–1374.
10. Albino A.P. (1987) The role of oncogenes in the pathogenesis of malignant melanoma. In: Nathanson L., ed. Basic and Clinical Aspects of Malignant Melanoma. Martinus Nijhoff, Boston, pp. 3–39.
11. Bale, S.J., Dracopoli, N.C., Tucker, M.A., Clark, W.H., Fraser, M.C., Stranger, B.Z., Green, P., Donis-Keller, H., Housman, D.E., Greene, M.H. (1989) Mapping the gene for hereditary cutaneous malignant melanoma-dysplastic nevus syndrome to chromosome 1p. N. Engl. J. Med. 320:1367–1372.
12. Trent, J.M., Thompson, F.H., Meyskens Jr., F.L. (1989) Identification of a recurring translocation site involving chromosome 6 in human malignant melanoma. Cancer Res. 49:420–423.
13. Dooley, T.P., Wilson, R.E., Jones, N.C., Hart, I.R. (1988) Polyoma middle T abrogates

TPA requirement of murine melanocytes and induces malignant melanoma. Oncogene 3:531–535.
14. Dotto, G.P., Moellmann, G., Ghosh, S., Edwards, M., Halaban, R. (1989) Transformation of murine melanocytes by basic fibroblast growth factor cDNA and oncogenes and selective suppression of the transformed phenotype in reconstituted cutaneous environment. J. Cell Biol. 109:3115–3128.
15. Halaban, R., Ghosh, S., Duray, P., Kirkwood, J.M., Lerner, A.B. (1986) Human melanocytes cultured from nevi and melanomas. J. Invest. Dermatol. 87:95–101.
16. Hecker, E. (1990) Phorbol esters from croton oil — Chemical nature and biological activities. Naturwissenschaften 54:282–284.
17. Collins, MKL, Rozengurt, E. (1982) Binding of phorbol esters to high-affinity sites on murine fibroblasts elicits a mitogenic response. J. Cell Physiol. 112:42–50.
18. Raick, A.N., Thumm, K., Chivers, B.R. (1972) Early effects of 12-O-tetradecanoyl-phorbol-13-acetate on the incorporation of tritiated precursor into DNA and the thickness of the interfollicular epidermis, and their relation to tumor promotion in mouse skin. Cancer Res. 32:1562–1568.
19. Nishizuka, Y. (1984) The role of protein kinase C in cell surface signal transduction and tumour promotion. Nature 308:693–698.
20. Nishizuka, Y. (1988) The molecular heterogeneity of protein kinase C and its implications for cellular regulation. Nature 334:661–665.
21. Creasey, A.A., Smith, H.S., Hackett, A.J., Fukuyama, K., Epstein, W.L. (1979) Biological properties of human melanoma cells in culture. In Vitro 15:342–350.
22. Tamaoki, T., Nomota, H., Takahashi, I., Kato, Y., Morimoto, M., Tomita, F. (1986) Staurosporine, a potent inhibitor of phospholipid/Ca^{++} dependent protein kinase. Biochem. Biophys. Res. Commun. 135:397–402.
23. Krauss, R.S., Housey, G.M., Johnson, M.D., Weinstein, I.B. (1989) Disturbances in growth control and gene expression in a C3H/10T1/2 cell line that stably overproduces protein kinase C. Oncogene 4:991–998.
24. Hsiao, W.L., Housey, G.M., Johnson, M.D., Weinstein, I.B. (1989) Cells that overproduce protein kinase C are more susceptible to transformation by an activated H-*ras* oncogene. Mol. Cell Biol. 9:2641–2647.
25. Halaban, R., Langdon, R., Birchall, N., Cuono, C., Baird, A., Scott, G., Moellmann, G., McGuire, J. (1988) Basic fibroblast growth factor from human keratinocytes is a natural mitogen for melanocytes. J. Cell Biol. 107:1611–1619.
26. Halaban, R., Ghosh, S., Baird, A. (1987) bFGF is the putative natural growth factor for human melanocytes. In Vitro Cell Dev. Biol. 23:47–52.
27. Herschman, H.R. (1989) Extracellular signals, transcriptional responses and cellular specificity. TIBS 14:455–458.
28. Coussens, L., Parker, P.J., Rhee., L., Yang-Feng, T.L., Chen., E., Waterfield, M.D., Francke, U., Ullrich, A. (1986) Multiple, distinct forms of bovine and human protein kinase C suggest diversity in cellular signaling pathways. Science 233:859–866.
29. Halaban, R. (1990) Responses of cultured melanocytes to defined growth factors. Pigment Cell Res. 1 (Suppl):18–26.
30. Pittlekow, M.R., Shipley, G.D. (1989) Serum-free culture of normal human melanocytes: Growth kinetics and growth factor requirements. J. Cell Physiol. 140:565–576.
31. Hicks, K., Friedman, B.A., Rosner, M.R. (1989) Basic and acidic fibroblast growth factors modulate the epidermal growth factor receptor by a protein kinase C-independent pathway. Biochem. Biolphys. Res. Commun. 164:796–803.
32. Paris, S, Chambard, J.-C., Pouseygeur, J. (1988) Tyrosine kinase-activating growth factors potentiate thrombin and AlF_4 induced phophoinositide breakdown in hamster fibroblasts. J. Biol. Chem. 263:12893–12900.
33. Herlyn., M., Clark, W.H., Rodeck, U., Mansianti, M.L., Jambrosic, J., Koprowski, H. (1987) Biology of tumor progression in human melanocytes. Lab. Invest. 56:461–473.
34. Rovera, G., Santoli, D., Damsky, C. (1979) Human promyelocytic leukemia cells in culture

differentiate into macrophage-like cells when treated with a phorbol diester. Proc. Natl. Acad. Sci. USA 76:2779–2783.

35. Pahlman, S., Odelstad, L., Larsson, E., Grotte, G., Nilsson, K. (1981) Phenotypic changes of human neuroblastoma cells in culture induced by 12-O-tetradecanoyl-phorbol-13-acetate. Int. J. Cancer 28:583–589.
36. Clemens, M.J., Tilleray, V.J., James, R., Gewert, D.R. (1988) Relationship of cellular oncogene expression to inhibition of growth and induction of differentiation of Daudi cells by interferons or TPA. J. Cell Biochem. 38:251–259.
37. Gescher, A., Reed, D.J. (1985) Characterization of the growth inhibition induced by tumor-promoting phorbol esters and of their receptor binding in A549 human lung carcinoma cells. Cancer Res. 45:4315–4321.
38. Yamada, S., Hirota, K., Chida, K., Kuroki, T. (1988) Inhibition of phorbol ester-caused induction of ornithine decarboxylase and tumor promotion in mouse skin by staurosporine, a potent inhibitor of protein kinase C. Biochem. Biophys. Res. Commun. 157:9–15.
39. Huang, F.L., Yoshida, Y., Cunha-Melo, J.R., Beaven, M.A., Huang, K.-P. (1989) Differential down-regulation of protein kinase C isozymes. J. Biol. Chem. 264:4238–4243.
40. Kreutter, D., Caldwell, A.B., Morin, M.J. (1985) Dissociation of protein kinase C activation from phorbol ester-induced maturation of HL-60 leukemia cells. J. Biol. Chem. 260:5979–5984.
41. Laughton, C.A., Dale, I.L., Gescher, A. (1989) Studies on bioactive compounds. 13. Synthesis and lack of growth-inhibitory properties of cyclo-1,2,4-triol 1,2-diesters, which resemble ring C of the phorbol ester molecule. J. Med. Chem. 32:428–433.
42. Angel, P., Imagawa, M., Chiu, R., Stein, B., Imbra, R.J., Rahmsdorf, H.J., Jonat, C., Herrlich, P., Karin, M. (1987) Phorbol ester-inducible genes contain a common cis element recognized by a TPA modulated trans-acting factor. Cell 49:729–739.
43. Halaban, R., Alfano, F.D. (1984) Selective elimination of fibroblasts from cultures of normal human melanocytes. In Vitro 20:447–450.
44. Chirgwin, J.M., Przybyla, A.E., MacDonald, R.J., Rutter, W.J. (1979) Isolation of biologically active ribonucleic acid from sources enriched in ribonuclease. Biochemistry 18:5294–5299.
45. Coppock, D.L., Pardee, A.B. (1987) Control of thymidine kinase mRNA during the cell cycle. Mol. Cell Biol. 7:2925–2932.

5. Regulation of growth and phenotype of normal human melanocytes in culture

Istvan T. Valyi-Nagy and Meenhard Herlyn

1. Introduction

The primary function of the melanocyte in the skin is to synthesize an optically dense and active pigment, melanin, to protect cells of the epidermis and dermis from the deleterious effects of ultraviolet (UV) light. The phenotypic characteristics of melanocytes have long been established. These are a) melanin production through the action of the cell-specific enzyme, tyrosinase; b) dendritic morphology; c) pigment donation via dendritic processes to adjacent keratinocytes; and d) unless specifically stimulated (i.e., by UV light), no detectable proliferation in situ. Despite the undetectable proliferation, a stable life-long 5–6:1 ratio is maintained between basal keratinocytes and melanocytes, suggesting a constant, controlled self-replication of epidermal pigmented cells. In this article we review the currently available data on maturation, growth requirements, and antigen expression of melanocytes and their interactions with keratinocytes.

2. Precursor stages in melanocyte maturation

Melanocytes are pigmented cells located in the basal layer of the epidermis, the infundibulum and the bulb of hair sheaths, the choroid of the eye, certain mucous membranes, and the leptomeninges. These neuroectoderm-derived cells leave the neural crest 2–3 weeks after fertilization. Subsequently, they migrate through the embryonal dermis to reach the epidermis by 8–10 weeks. These immature precursor cells, *melanoblasts*, are devoid of active melanin production and do not actively produce pigment until after birth, with the exception of the slightly pigmented areas of the nipples and the genitalia. Ultrastructurally, these cells possess premelanosomes (grade I and II melanosomes; melanosome precursors lacking melanin) but do not exhibit tyrosinase activity [1]. The pathway of maturation of melanocytes, as summarized in Table 1, is still unclear. Experimental evidence to delineate each maturation stage of melanocytes remains incomplete, but it appears that melanoblasts undergo at least two precursor stages before maturing. Inter-

L. Nathanson (ed.), MELANOMA RESEARCH: GENETICS, GROWTH FACTORS, METASTASES, AND ANTIGENS.

Table 1. Maturation of melanocytes

Cell type	Phenotype	Location
Melanoblast ↓↑ ↓↑	?	Migrating from neural crest
Early premelanocyte ↓ ↑ ↓ ↑	Round, noncharacteristic; premelanosomes; tyrosinase activity – (a) pigmentation – proliferation (b)	Fetal dermis; outer sheath of hair follicle; adult dermis (?)
Intermediate or late premelanocyte ↓ ↓	Uni- or bipolar premelanosomes tyrosinase activity – (a) pigmentation ± proliferation (b)	Fetal dermis; adult dermis (?); infundibulum of hair follicle
Melanocyte	Bi-, tripolar, or multidendritic; premelanosomes and melanosomes; tyrosinase activity + pigmentation + proliferation (b)	Basal layers of skin; infundibulum and bulb of hair follicle; (eye/ mucous membranes, leptomeninges)

Modified from refs. 1, 2, 4, and 5.
Tyrosinase activity (a) and proliferation (b) can be specifically modulated by culture conditions and forced regeneration.
——→ maturation.
----→ reversion.

mediate cell types, *premelanocytes*, can be isolated, cultured, and cloned from neonatal human skin [2]. These cells are unpigmented or slightly pigmented, and contain grade I and II melanosomes (premelanosomes). The vast majority of these cells are tyrosinase negative; however, activation of tyrosinase and pigmentation can be achieved by elevating the pH of culturing medium from 6.8 to 7.4 and supplementing the medium with 1 mM tyrosine, the precursor of melanin. Following these manipulations, pigmentation of these unpigmented or barely pigmented clones occurs gradually [2]. The initially unstable, then stable, activation of melanin synthesis has led to the concept of gradual commitment of these cells in their maturation pathway [3,4]. Benett hypothesized that stable commitment occurs when melanocytes become pigmented. Analysis of clones of human melanocytes and murine melanoma cells showed that the likelihood of reversion from more-pigmented cells to a less-pigmented cell type decreased with the increasing degree of pigmentation [3]. Reversion was never observed in well-pigmented clones; thus, these cells could be considered as stably committed cells. Reversion of human premelanocyte clones, however, could only be observed when cells were very lightly pigmented, whereas reversion of murine melanoma clones exhibiting divergent degrees of pigmentation was frequently noticed [3]. In conclusion, the gradual commitment of melanocytic cells parallels the development of pigmentation. Maturation is associated with a falling probability of reversion and is complete when the likelihood of reversion approaches zero [4].

The putative equivalents of the premelanocytes in vivo can be found in the outer sheath of the hair follicles. In the hair follicles, pigmented melanocytes are characteristically located in the wall of the pilary canal (infundibulum) and in the pigmented portion of the hair bulb. Conversely, the outer sheath of the middle portion of the follicle contains amelanotic melanocytes. It is suggested that these cells, under the stimuli of epidermal regeneration and/or following UV irradiation, undergo serial divisions, migrate up toward the infundibular portion of the follicle, and gradually mature into dendritic, pigmented melanocytes. It is also believed that, when the stimulus subsides, these cells revert into inactivity [5].

Mature melanocytes are multidendritic pigmented cells that are located mainly in the basal layer of the epidermis. These cells are tyrosinase positive and produce pigment through the action of the tyrosinase enzyme. These cells contain melanosomes of all (I–IV) stages of maturation and transport pigment to adjacent keratinocytes.

3. Growth requirements of normal human melanocytes in vitro

The development of meticulous isolation methods and special culture media for selective growth and long-term maintenance of melanocytes has been a major basic contribution to our understanding of pigment cell biology. Attempts at isolating and growing human melanocytes had been made for almost 30 years [6–10]. It was only in 1982 when pure cultures of normal human melanocytes could be reproducibly established to yield large quantities of cells for biological, biochemical, and molecular analysis. Eisinger and Marko [11] found that a tumor promoter, phorbol 12-myristate-13-acetate (PMA), and an intracellular cyclic adenosine 3′,5′monophosphate (cAMP) enhancer, cholera toxin, were strong mitogens for melanocytes. The first report on a natural melanocyte mitogen was provided by Gilchrest et al. [12], who used bovine hypothalamus extracts and cholera toxin for melanocyte culture. The recent, rapid development of tissue culture methods has led to the advent of effective, standardized procedures for the culture of human epidermal melanocytes.

Deletion of serum and brain tissue extracts from medium has led to the delineation of four groups of chemically defined melanocyte mitogens: a) peptide growth factors, b) calcium and cation binding proteins, c) enhancers of intracellular levels of cAMP, and d) activators of protein kinase C. Ultraviolet light (UV-B) appears to be the only physical mitogen with a known growth stimulatory effect [13–16]. Table 2 summarizes the factors that modulate the growth stimulatory of melanocytes in culture.

Table 2. Factors that modulate melanocyte growth and/or morphology in culture

Name	Main type of action	Reference
Polypeptide growth factors		
bFGF	Growth promotion	17
Insulin/IGF-1	Growth promotion	21
EGF/TGFα	Growth promotion[a]	20–22
TGFβ	Growth inhibition	22
Calcium and cation binding proteins		
Ca^{2+} (1.0–2.0 mM)	Growth promotion	23
Tyrosinase (Cu^{2+})	Growth promotion	23
Ceruloplasmin (Cu^{2+})	Growth promotion	23
Transferrin (Fe^{2+})	Growth promotion	23
Activators of adenylate cyclase[b]		
α-MSH	Growth promotion	23
FSH	Growth promotion	23
Cholera toxin	Growth promotion	11
Forskolin	Growth promotion	23
Isobutyl methylxanthine (IBMX)	Growth promotion	26
Activators of protein kinase C		
TPA	Growth promotion	11
PDBu	Growth promotion	28
Miscellaneous compounds		
Dibutyryl cAMP	Growth promotion/morphology	29
Histamine	Morphology	30
$1{,}25(OH)_2$ vitamin-D_3/ $25(OH)$ vitamin-D_3	Morphology/growth promotion?	35
Prostaglandin $F_{2a}(PGF_{2a})$ $E_2(PGE_2)$	Growth promotion/morphology	23,24
Extracellular matrix (ECM)	Morphology/growth modulation?	36
Physical agents		
Ultraviolet light (UV-B, UV-C)	Growth promotion/morphology	13,14

[a] Only during the initial passage of melanocytes.
[b] Intracellular enhancement of cAMP has not been demonstrated on human melanocytes.

3.1. Peptide growth factors. The main growth-promoting polypeptide in bovine brain (hypothalamus) and pituitary extracts is basic fibroblast growth factor (bFGF) [17,18]. Basic FGF can exert its stimulatory effect only in combination with either cAMP-enhancing components or activators of protein kinase C. Insulinlike growth factor-I (IGF-I) and insulin share a similar growth-promoting effect, since they bind to the same cell surface receptor. It has been shown, however, that the affinity of IGF-I for this receptor on melanoma cells is approximately 100-fold higher [19]. Epidermal growth factor (EGF) supports the growth of melanocytes during the initial passage, but is not mitogenic for established cultures [20,21]. Transforming growth factor-alpha (TGF-α) has a similar, if not identical, effect. TGF-β, on the other hand, is an inhibitor of melanocyte growth [22].

3.2. Calcium and cation binding proteins

Ca^{2+} is an important cation in melanocyte growth media. Its optimal concentration is 1.0–2.0 mM. Reduction of calcium concentration in medium to 0.03 mM reduces cell growth by approximately 50% [23]. Cation binding proteins, such as tyrosinase (copper), ceruloplasmin (copper), or transferrin (iron), are mitogenic for melanocytes [23].

3.3. Compounds that enhance the intracellular level of cAMP

There are a great variety of compounds of diverse origin that have been described to be mitogens for melanocytes in cultures [23]. Alpha-melanocyte stimulating hormone (α-MSH) is a very strong mitogen in chemically defined melanocyte growth medium for human melanocytes, but the mechansims of action are not clear. Conversely, beta-melanocyte stimulating hormone (β-MSH) probably has no effect on human melanocytes [24]. Forskolin and follicle-stimulating hormone, after increasing the intracellular level of cAMP, also increase the binding of insulin to the cells [25].

Cholera toxin, tetanus toxin, and pertussis toxin probably also augment intracellular cAMP levels, however, enhancement of intracellular cAMP has not been unequivocally proven in cultured melanocytes. Cholera toxin is commonly added to melanocyte media [11,12,26] and the B subunit is most effective [23]. It has also been shown that GM1 monosialoganglioside is the receptor for cholera toxin that can act as a bimodal regulator of cellular growth, generating either negative or positive signals for cell growth [27].

3.4. Protein kinase C activator phorbol esters

Protein kinase C activating phorbol esters are very strong mitogens for melanocytes. 12-0-tetradeconoyl-phorbol-13-acetate (TPA) is lipophilic, so it cannot be removed from the cells by simple washing. 20-oxo-phorbol-12-13-dibutyrate (PDBu) is a similar, but more hydrophilic, derivative [28]. Besides their mitogenic effect, phorbol esters also modulate the morphology of melanocytes to a high degree (see below). Withdrawal of phorbol ester from melanocyte growth medium induces a 'fibroblastoid' morphologic change (Figure 1B) and a grossly decreased growth rate. This change is reversible on the condition that the growth medium is replenished with phorbol ester within 14 days. Thus, these compounds are necessary not only for maintaining cell proliferation, but also for the maintenance of the characteristic bi- or tripolar phenotype (Figure 1A) [11].

3.5. Miscellaneous compounds with impact on melanocyte growth and/ or morphology

Dibutyryl cAMP (dbcAMP) is a very strong inducer of dendrite formation (Figure 1C). The number of dendritic process increased about tenfold within

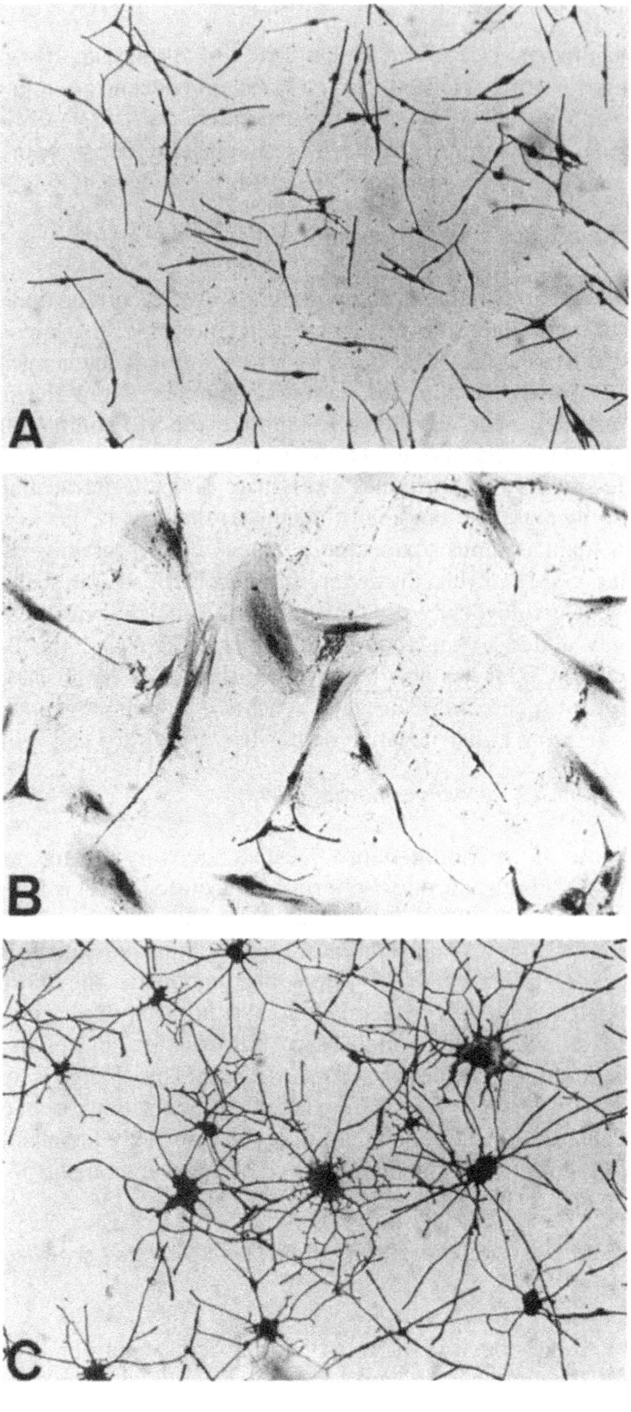
A
B
C

4–6 days of dbcAMP [23]. This morphologic effect is reversible; melanocytes reassume their bi- or tripolar morphology 4–8 days after the removal of dbcAMP from medium. dbcAMP also has a growth-promoting effect when used together with cholera toxin [29].

Histamine, produced in the skin by mast cells, is also stimulatory for cultured melanocytes [30]. In a dose-dependent fashion, histamine increases both the amount of tyrosinase and the size of melanocytes, and cells also become more dendritic. These changes can already be observed 6 hours after supplementing the medium with histamine.

1,25-dihydroxyvitamin D_3 (1,25$(OH)_2D_3$) and 25-hydroxyvitamin D_3 (25$(OH)D_3$) are the active derivatives of vitamin D_3. The precursors of this hormone are synthesized in the basal layer of the skin upon exposure to UV light. Normal human melanocytes, melanoma cells, and keratinocytes have the biochemical capacity to convert vitamin D_3 into its active hydroxylated metabolites [31–33]. Topical treatment of mice with cholecalciferol or 1,25$(OH)_2D_3$ increase the number of pigmented cells. This phenomenon is due either to the reactivation of residing melanocytes or to a direct mitogenic effect. The effect of the topical treatment can be blocked by simultaneous oral treatment with indomethacin. This suggests that prostaglandins, probably produced by surrounding keratinocytes, act as modulators and/or mediators to pigmented cells. In fact, prostaglandin F_{2a} was shown to have a strong stimulatory effect on melanocytes, using chemically defined media [23]. Treating cells with prostaglandin E_2, but not E_1, results in only morphological changes [34]. In cultured human melanocytes, however, 1,25$(OH)_2D_3$, and to a lesser extent 25$(OH)D_3$, cause a marked decrease of tyrosinase activity. The differences between the results obtained from animal experiments and in-vitro studies might be due to the lack of keratinocytes and Langerhans cells in the culture system, which may be the sources of other, coacting mediators. It has also been shown that human melanocytes in culture express cell surface receptors to vitamin D_3. The isolated receptor molecule was found to migrate in the 53-kD region [35].

Human epidermal melanocytes cultured on extracellular matrix (ECM)-coated plastic surfaces develop flatter and larger cell bodies, and present with an increased melanin production. Pigmented human melanoma cells are not affected by the presence of ECM [36].

Melanocytes from newborn foreskin grown in the presence of insulin, EGF, pituitary extract, fetal calf serum, and TPA grow at doubling times of 1–4 days for 40–60 doublings. Heavily pigmented cells may senesce after 20–30 doublings. Dendricity may increase at higher passage levels. Normal

Figure 1. Melanocytes grown on a medium supplemented with bFGF (pituitary extract), serum, and phorbol esters. Pigmented cells have slim cellular bodies with two to four dendrites. A. Morphology of melanocytes 14 days after phorbol ester was omitted from medium: cell bodies are enlarged and flat; dendricity is decreased ('fibroblastoid' changed). B. Melanocytes treated with dibutyryl cAMP exhibit an increased tendency for dendrite formation C.

melanocytes have a diploid karyotype and are nontumorigenic in athymic nude mice. These cells do not proliferate anchorage independently in soft agar [20].

4. Morphology and antigenic phenotype of melanocytes

4.1. Morphology

Normal melanocytes, grown in W489 medium supplemented with 2% FCS, TPA, pituitary extract, insulin, and 2mM $CaCl_2$, exhibit a bi- or tripolar morphology, with varying degrees of cytoplasmic pigment (Figure 1A and group 1 in Table 3). Ultrastructurally, these cells contain melanosomes from all stages of maturation. Melanocytes grown in PBDu- instead of TPA-containing medium have a similar morphology, but they are less dendritic, appear longer, and continue to divide, but at a slower rate. If TPA is removed at passge 5 from medium, cells slow in their growth rate, the morphology becomes flat, and the pigmentation disappears (Figure 1B and group 1 in Table 3). By passage 8, cells senesce and cannot be passaged further. Cells grown in the presence of dbcAMP (in addition of TPA) develop multiple dendrities (Figure 1C). The dendrite formation begins after 2–5 days and is reversible when dbcAMP is removed from medium. If melanocytes are established in medium without TPA, they grow at doubling times of 3–6 days for the first 2–3 passages and then they senesce by passage 5 (subgroup A

Table 3. Phenotype of melanocytes isolated from newborn foreskin[a]

		Growth			Morphology[b]			Pigmentation		
Group	Culture condition	p.1	p.5	p.8	p.1	p.5	p.8	p.1	p.5	p.8
1.	TPA	+++	+++	+++	D	D	D	+++	+++	+++
	No TPA p.5 ↳		↳	0		↳	F		↳	0
2.	No TPA (subgroup A)	+++	+	0	S	F	F	+	0	0
	TPA p.1 ↳[c]	↳	+++		↳	D			++	
	TPA p.5 ↳		↳	0		↳	F		↳	0
	No TPA (subgroup B)	+++	+++	+++	S	S	S	0	0	0
	TPA p.5 ↳		↳	+++		↳	S/D		↳	+
3.	Coculture with keratinocytes	++	++		D	D		+	+	
	TPA p.1 ↳	↳	+++	+++	↳	D	D	↳	++	++

[a] All cultures were maintained in same base medium: W489 medium with insulin, EGF, 40 μg/ml bovine pituitary extract, and 2% FCS.
[b] S = spindle; F = flat, polygonal; D = dendritic, + → +++ = degree of growth or pigmentation; 0 = no growth or > 14 days doubling and no pigmentation.
[c] Addition of TPA to medium at passage 1, followed by continued presence of TPA in medium.

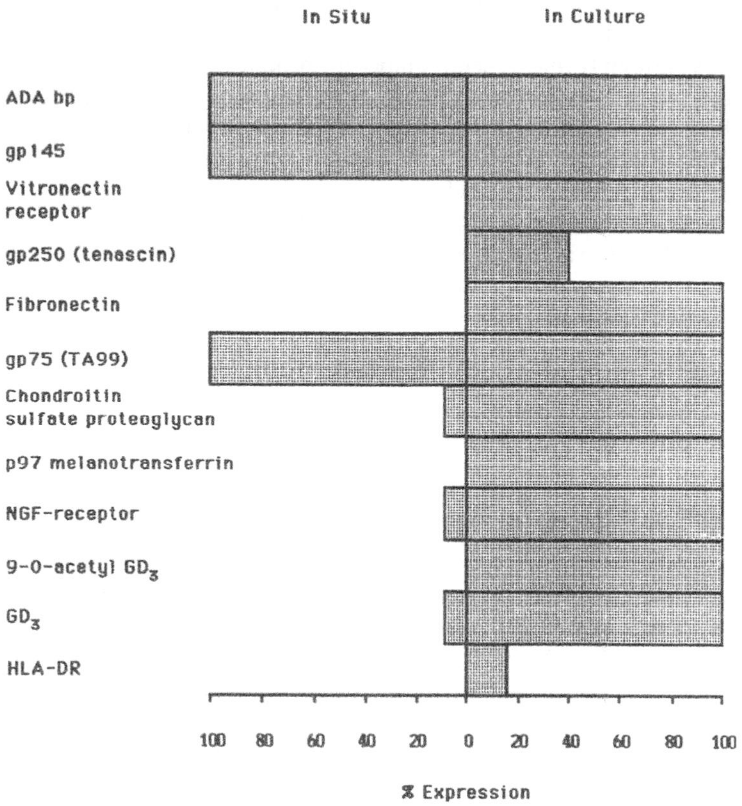

Figure 2. Expression of antigens on melanocytes in situ (left panel) and in culture (right panel). Bars indicate the percentage of specimen and cultures expressing antigens as tested with MAbs. Results with cultured melanocytes are show with TPA-containing medium at passages 2–20, with the exception of gp145. gp145 is expressed more strongly on melanocytes cultured in the absence of TPA.

of group 2 in Table 3). Addition of TPA induces the bipolar, pigmented phenotype only when added to the medium at passage 1, not at passage 5. A subgroup of melanocytes, representing approximately 15% of the specimens, preserves a stable phenotype when established in the absence of TPA (subgroup B of group 2 in Table 3). These cells continue to proliferate after passage 5, remain responsive to TPA, and are of spindle morphology and nonpigmented [21].

In coculture with keratinocytes, melanocytes assume a dendritic morphology that is similar to that in TPA-containing medium (Figure 3 and group 3 in Table 3). Cocultured melanocytes continue to be responsive to TPA, even after keratinocytes (due to the presence of TPA in medium) have terminally differentiated and dissappeared.

4.2. Antigenic phenotype of normal melanocytes

Only few attempts have been made to produce monoclonal antibodies (MAbs) to normal melanocytes [37,21]. On the other hand, extensive studies have been done to characterize the antigenic phenotype of malignant melanoma cells [38]. Figure 2 summarizes the expression of melanocyte-associated antigens in situ and in vitro. Cultured melanocytes share with melanoma cells the expression of a variety of cell surface antigens, including p97 melanotransferrin, vitronectin receptor, gangliosides GD_3 and 9-0-acetyl GD_3, and chondroitin sulfate proteoglycan [21]. In situ, however, these antigens are not expressed by melanocytes [39]. Weak expression on melanocytes in situ of the receptor for nerve growth factor contrasts to strong expression on cultured cells. The reason for this divergent antigenic phenotype in culture and in situ is not known, but it is assumed that cultured cells, due to their rapid proliferation, acquire the enhanced expression of melanoma-associated antigens. The expression of these antigens on melanocytes, on the other hand, does not appear to reflect a 'transformed' phenotype.

Melanocytes in situ and in culture also express antigens that are not found on melanoma cells. These include adenosine deaminase binding protein (ADA bp) [40] and gp145, detected by antibody 487 [20]. Potentially, the group of antigens referred to as 'suppressor antigens' is much larger, and they may play important roles in the pathogenesis of melanoma development.

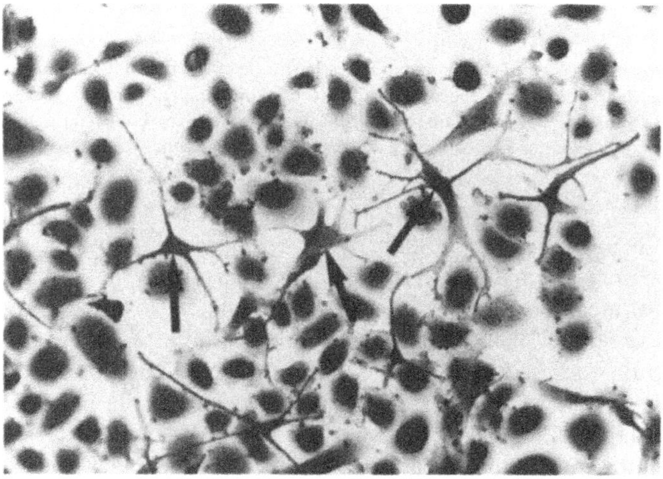

Figure 3. In monolayer cocultures with keratinocytes, melanocytes (arrows) survive for a prolonged time without adding phorbol esters and adenylate cyclase inducers to medium. Calcium concentration in this medium is low (0.03 mM), as opposed to the 2.0 mM calcium concentration required for optimal growth of melanocytes. Melanocytes preserve their mature, dendritic phenotype and contact adjacent keratinocytes with their dendrites.

Table 4. Expression of cell surface antigens on melanocytes

		NGF receptor			gp145K		
Group	Cultured condition	p.1	p.5	p.8	p.1	p.5	p.8
1.	TPA	++	+++	+++	0	0	+
	No TPA p.5 ↳		↳	+		↳	++
2.	A. No TPA	++++	0			+++	
	TPA p.5 ↳		↳	0		↳	++
	B. No TPA	+++	+++	+++	0	+	+

+ → +++ = increasing degree of expression; 0 = no expression.

As shown in Table 4, the antigenic phenotype of cultured melanocytes varies depending on the culture conditions and changes with the morphological phenotype (for comparison, see also Table 3). At the onset of culture, all melanocytes express a variety of melanoma-associated antigens, regardless of whether or not TPA is added to medium. However, after five passages in medium without TPA, expression of the NGF receptor disappears, whereas gp145 is strongly expressed (group 1 in Table 4). Cells cultured in a TPA-containing medium (group 1 in Table 4) and a rare variant of cells without the addition of TPA (group 2B in Table 4) strongly express NGF receptor throughout their lifespan.

5. regulation of growth and phenotype of melanocytes by normal human keratinocytes in vitro

The symbiosis of the three major cell types in the epidermis, i.e., keratinocytes, melanocytes, and Langerhans cells, follows strict rules. Keratinocytes of the basal or germinative layer constantly divide, and, while moving upwards within the epidermis, undergo a well-characterized, gradual differentiation pathway. Melanocytes, on the other hand, never leave the basal layer, and, unless specifically stimulated, do not divide.

For optimal growth in culture, melanocytes require bFGF, phorbol esters, intracellular cAMP enhancers, and 2 mM calcium. In contrast to this, keratinocytes have strikingly divergent growth requirements (Table 5). Phorbol esters induce growth arrest and terminal differentiation of keratinocytes [41]. Serum and calcium also induce their terminal differentiation [42,43]. Both cell types need bFGF in growth medium, but EGF is required only by kertinocytes.

In serum-free keratinocyte growth medium, melanocytes do not survive. When cocultured with normal human keratinocytes in this medium, melanocytes survive for a prolonged time [44,45]. It has also been shown that in these cocultures melanocytes maintain their mature dendritic phenotype, contact surrounding keratinocytes with their dendrites, and donate pigment in a similar fashion to that in vivo (Figure 3) [45].

Table 5. Growth requirements of normal human melanocytes and keratinocytes

	Melanocytes	Keratinocytes
bFGF (pituitary extract)	Required	Required
Insulin/IGF-1	Required	Required
TPA (phorbol esters)	Required	Terminal differentiation
2 mM Ca^{2+}	Required	Terminal differentiation
EGF	Only initially	Required

In three-dimensional epidermal reconstructs, keratinocytes differentiate into three layers that morphologically and antigenically resemble the basal, spinous, and cornified layers of the intact skin. The vast majority of melanocytes, cocultured with keratinocytes in these skin equivalents, are located within the basal layer of the epidermis, maintain their dendritic phenotype, and donate pigment to surrounding keratinocytes (Figure 4) [45]. Under these experimental conditions, the ratio between epidermal cells and melanocytes remains constant [46]. Only cocultured epidermal keratinocytes, but not oral epidermal cells, had regulatory effects on melanocytes [47].

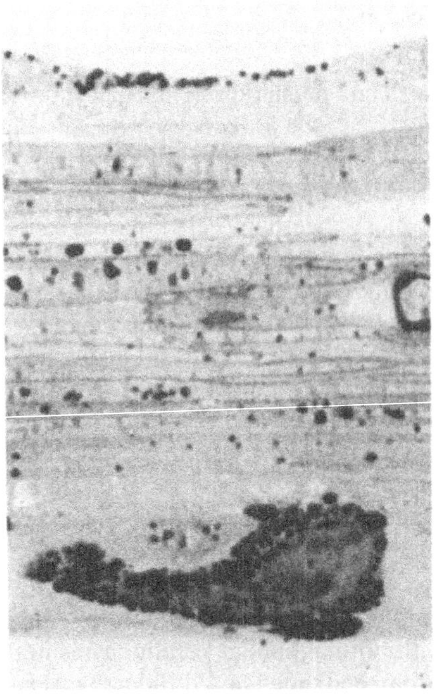

Figure 4. The majority of melanocytes in three-dimensional epidermal reconstructs are located within the basal layer of the epidermis. In this environment, pigmented cells remain viable for up to 30 days and donate pigment to surrounding epidermal cells.

Table 6. Growth factor, cytokine, and hormone production of undifferentiated keratinocytes in culture

Product	Activity	Reference
Basic fibroblast growth factor (bFGF)	Autocrine and paracrine growth stimulator	44
Transforming growth factor-alpha (TGF-α)	Autocrine and paracrine growth stimulator	50
Transforming growth factor-beta (TGF-β)	Autocrine and paracrine growth inhibitor Stimulator of keratinocyte motility and fibronectin secretion	56,57
Interleukin-1 (IL-1)/epidermal cell-derived thymocyte activating factor (ETAF) (produced in inactive form, site of inactivation is unknown)	T-cell activator, induces cytokine release from other cells, induces collagen and collagenase production of fibroblasts, promotes melanocyte pigmentation, promotes antigen presentation by Langerhans cells	51,52
Interleukin-3 (IL-3)	Cofactor in T-cell and mast-cell activation	52
Interferon-alpha (INF-α)	Differentiation inducer, inhibits proliferation, mediator in immunologic reactions	53
Interferon-beta (INF-β)/ interleukin (IL-6)	Stimulator of B-cells and keratinocytes	54,55
Epidermal cell-derived natural killer cell activating factor (ENKAF)	NK-cell activation	52
Granulocyte-monocyte colony stimulating factor (GM-CSF)/ keratinocyte-derived T-cell growth factor (KTGF)	T-cell and granulocyte/monocyte activation	58
Vitamin D_3 1,25-dihydroxyvitamin D_3 ($1{,}25(OH)_2D_3$); 25-hydroxyvitamin D_3 ($25(OH)D_3$)	Systemic effect on calcium and phosphate metabolism, autocrine and paracrine growth modulation of epidermal cells (?)	32
Low molecular weight keratinocyte-derived substance (< 500 kD)	Modulation of melanocyte morphology	49
High molecular weight keratinocyte-derived substance	Growth promotion of melanocytes	49

The fact that melanocytes in coculture with keratinocytes remain viable and assume a mature phenotype and function without the presence of their standard in-vitro mitogens, i.e., phorbol esters and adenylate cyclase activators, suggests the production of maturation factors by keratinocytes. Basic FGF, produced by epidermal keratinocytes, is certainly one of the growth-modulating factors for melanocytes [17,44]. Keratinocyte/melanocyte contact also appears to be required for the interactions of these two cell types [44–48]. Recently it has been suggested that keratinocyte-derived substances of high molecular weight stimulate melanocyte growth, while low molecular weight compounds (< 500 kD) promote dendricity and melanization [49].

These studies demonstrate that keratinocytes, in vitro, and most likely also in vivo, release factors that regulate and/or modulate the growth and differentiation of melanocytes. The keratinocyte, the predominant cell type of the epidermis, has an enormously broad variety of metabolic capabilities, i.e., vitamin and hormone, as well as growth factor and cytokine production. (For summary and references, see Table 6.) The majority of these factors have an impact on growth, morphology, and/or antigen expression of melanocytes in culture. Conversely, very little is known about the effect of Langerhans cells on epidermal homeostasis. In addition, epidermal cells are under the constant surveillance of the neuroendocrine system. Normal human melanocytes also have the ability to recognize and respond to signals generated by and/or transmitted via the extracellular matrix (see Table 2). This ability appears to be altered or absent in melanoma cells [36].

References

1. Hirobe, T. (1982) Genes involved in regulating the melanocyte and melanoblast-melanocyte populations in the epidermis of newborn mouse skin. J. Exp. Zool. 223:257–264.
2. Bennett, D.C., Bridges, K., McKay, I.A. (1985) Clonal separation of mature melanocytes from premelanocytes in a diploid human cell strain: Spontaneous and induced pigmentation of premelanocytes. J. Cell. Sci. 77:167–183.
3. Bennett, D.C. (1983) Differentiation in mouse melanoma cells: Initial reversibility and an on-off stochastic model. Cell 34:445–453.
4. Bennett, D.C. (1989) Mechanisms of differentiation in melanoma cells and melanocytes. Environ. Health Persp. 80:49–59.
5. Staricco, R.G. (1963) Amelanotic melanocytes in the outer sheath of the human hair follicle and their role in the pigmentation of regenerated epidermis. Ann. N.Y. Acad. Sci. 100:239–255.
6. Hu, F., Staricco, R.J., Pinkus, H., Fosnaugh, R. (1957) Human melanocytes in tissue culture. J. Invest. Dermatol. 28:15–32.
7. Karasek, M., Charlton, M.E. (1980) Isolation and growth of normal human skin melanocytes. Clin. Res. 28:570A.
8. Kitano, Y. (1976) Stimulation by melanocyte stimulating hormone and dibutyryl adenosine 3′,5′-cyclic monophosphate of DNA synthesis in human melanocytes in vitro. Arch. Derm. Res. 257:47–52.
9. Mayer, T.C. (1982) The control of embryonic pigment cell proliferation in culture by cyclic AMP. Dev. Biol. 94:509–614.
10. Wilkins, L.M., Szabo, G.C. (1981) Use of mycostatin-supplemented media to establish pure epidermal melanocyte culture (abstract). J. Invest. Dermatol. 76:332.
11. Eisinger, M., Marko, O. (1982) Selective proliferation of normal human melanocytes in vitro in the presence of phorbol ester and cholera toxin. Proc. Natl. Acad. Sci. USA 79:2018–2022.
12. Gilchrest, B.A., Vrabel, M.A., Flynn, E., Szabo, G. (1984) Selective cultivation of human melanocytes from newborn and adult epidermis. J. Invest. Dermatol. 83:370–376.
13. Rosdahl, I.K., Szabo, G. (1978) Mitotic activity of epidermal melanocytes in UV-irradiated mouse skin. J. Invest. Dermatol. 70:143–148.
14. Friedman, P.S., Gilchrest, B.A. (1987) Ultraviolet radiation directly induces pigment

production by cultured human melanocytes. J. Cell. Physiol. 133:88–94.
15. Libow, L.F., Scheide, S., DeLeo, V.A. (1988) Ultraviolet radiation acts ac an independent mitogen for normal human melanocytes in culture. Pigment Cell Res. 1:397–401.
16. Stierner, U., Rosdahl, I., Augustsson, A., Kagedal, B. (1989) UVB irradiation induces melanocyte increase in both exposed and shielded human skin. J. Invest. Dermatol. 92:561–564.
17. Halaban, R., Ghosh, S., Baird, A. (1987) bFGF is the putative natural growth factor for human melanocytes. In Vitro 23:47–52.
18. Halaban, R., Kwon, B.S., Ghosh, S., Delli Bovi, P., Baird, A. (1988) bFGF as an autocrine growth factor for human melanomas. Oncogene Res. 3:177–186.
19. Rodeck, U., Herlyn, M., Menssen, H.D., Furlanetto, R.W., Koprowski, H. (1987) Metastatic but not primary melanoma cell lines grow in vitro independently of exogenous growth factors. Int. J. Cancer 40:687–690.
20. Herlyn, M., Rodeck, U., Mancianti, M.L., Cardillo, F.M., Lang, A., Ross, A.H., Jambrosic, J., Koprowski, H. (1987) Expression of melanoma-associated antigens in rapidly dividing human melanocytes in culture. Cancer Res. 47:3057–3061.
21. Herlyn, M., Clark, W.H., Rodeck, U., Mancianti, M.L., Jambrosic, J., Koprowski, H. (1987) Biology of tumor progression in human melanocytes. Lab. Invest. 56:461–474.
22. Pittelkow, M.R., Shipley, G.D. (1989) Serum-free culture of normal human melanocytes: Growth kinetics and growth factor requirements. J. Cell. Physiol. 140:565–576.
23. Herlyn, M., Mancianti, M.L., Jambrosic, J., Bolen, J.B., Koprowski, H. (1988) Regulatory factors that determine growth and phenotype of normal human melanocytes. Exp. Cell Res. 179:322–331.
24. Abdel-Malek, Z.A. (1988) Endocrine factors as effectors of integumental pigmentation. In: Dermatologic Clinics, Vol. 6. W.B. Saunders, Philadelphia, pp. 175–184.
25. Adashi, E.Y., Resnick, C.E., Svoboda, M.E., Van Wyk, J.J. (1986) Follicle-stimulating hormone enhances somatomedin C binding to cultured rat granulosa cells. J. Biol. Chem. 261(9):3923–3926.
26. Halaban, R., Pomeranz, S.H., Marshall, S., Lambert, D.T., Lerner, A.B. (1983) Regulation of tyrosinase in human melanocytes grown in culture. J. Cell Biol. 97:480–488.
27. Spiegel, S., Fishman, P.H. (1987) Gangliosides as bimodal regulators of cell growth. Proc. Natl. Acad. Sci. USA 84:141–145.
28. Niedel, J.E., Blackshear, P.J. (1986) Protein kinase C. In: Phosphoinositides and Receptor Mechanisms, Alan R. Liss, New York, pp. 47-88.
29. Halaban, R. (1988) Responses of cultured melanocytes to defined growth factors. Pigm. Cell. Res. Suppl. 1:18–26.
30. Tomita, Y., Kazuhisa, M., Hachiro, T. (1988) Stimulatory effect of histamine on normal human melanocytes in vitro. Tohoku J. Exp. Med. 155:209–210.
31. Frankel, T.L., Mason, R.S., Hersey, E., Posen, S. (1983) The synthesis of vitamin D metabolites by human melanoma cells. J. Clin. Endocrinol. Metab. 57:627–631.
32. Bikle, D.D., Nemanic, M.K., Gee, E., Elias, P. (1986) 1,25-dihydroxyvitamin D_3 production by human keratinocytes. J. Clin. Invest. 78:557–566.
33. Tomita, Y., Torinuki, W., Tagami, H. (1988) Stimulation of human melanocytes by vitamin D_3 possibly mediates skin pigmentation after sun exposure. J. Invest. Dermatol, 90:882–884.
34. Tomita, Y., Iwamoto, M., Masuda, T., Tagami, H. (1987) Stimulatory effect of prostaglandin E_2 on the configuration of normal human melanocytes in vitro. J. Invest. Dermatol. 89:299–301.
35. Abdel-Malek, Z.A., Ross, R., Trinkle, L., Swope, V., Pike, J.W., Nordlund, J.J. (1988) Hormonal effects of vitamin D_3 on epidermal melanocytes. J. Cell. Physiol. 136:273–280.
36. Ranson, M., Posen, S., Mason, R.S. (1988) Extracellular matrix modulates the function of human melanocytes but not melanoma cells. J. Cell. Physiol. 136:281–288.
37. Houghton, A.N., Eisinger, M., Albino, A.P., Cairncross, J.G., Old, L.J. (1982) Surface antigens of melanocytes and melanomas: Markers of melanocyte differentiation and mela-

noma subsets. J. Exp. Med. 156:1755–1766.
38. Herlyn, M., Koprowski, H. (1988) Melanoma antigens: Immunological and biological characterization and clinical significance. Ann. Rev. Immunol. 6:283–308.
39. Elder, D.E., Rodeck, U., Thurin, J., Cardillo, F., Clark, W.H., Stewart, R., Herlyn, M. (1989) Antigenic profile of tumor progression stages in human melanocyte nevi and melanomas. Cancer Res. 49:5091–5096.
40. Houghton, A.N., Albino, A.P., Cordon-Cardo, C., Davis, L.J., Eisinger, M. (1988) Cell surface antigens of human melanocytes and melanoma: Expression of adenosine deaminase binding protein is extinguished with melanocyte transformation. J. Exp. Med. 167:197–212.
41. Willie, J.J., Pittelkow, M.R., Scott, R.E. (1985) Normal and transformed human prokerantinocytes express divergent effects of a tumor promoter on cell cycle-mediated control of proliferation and differentiation. Carcinogenesis. 6:1181–1187.
42. Boyce, S.T., Harn, R.G. (1983) Calcium-regulated differentiation of normal human epidermal keratinocytes in chemically defined clonal culture and serum-free serial culture. J. Invest. Dermatol. 81:33s-40s.
43. Pittelkow, M.R., Scott, R.E. (1986) New techniques for the in vitro culture of human skin keratinocytes and perspectives on their use for grafting of patients with extensive burns. Mayo Clin. Proc. 61:771–777.
44. Halaban, R., Langdon, R., Birchall, N., Cuono, C., Baird, A., Scott, G., Moellmann, G., McGuire, J. (1988) Basic fibroblast growth factor from human keratinocytes in a natural mitogen for melanocytes. J. Cell Biol. 107:1611–1619.
45. Valyi-Nagy, I.T., Murphy, G.F., Mancianti, M.L., Whitaker, D., Herlyn, M. (1990) Phenotypes and interactions of human melanocytes and keratinocytes in an epidermal reconstruction model. Lab. Invest., in press.
46. DeLuca, M., Franzi, A.T., D'Anna, F., Zicca, A., Albanese, E., Bondanza, S., Cancedda, R. (1988) Coculture of human keratinocytes and melanocytes: Differentiated melanocytes are physiologically organized in the basal layer of the cultured epithelium. Eur. J. Cell Biol. 46:176–180.
47. DeLuca, M., D'Anna, F., Bondanza, S., Franzi, A.T., Cancedda, R. (1988) Human epithelial cells induce human melanocyte growth in vitro but only skin keratinocytes regulate its proper differentiation in the absence of dermis. J. Cell. Biol. 107:1919–1926.
48. Bertaux, B., Moliere, P., Moreno, G., Courtalon, A., Masse, J.M., Dubertet, L. (1988) Growth of melanocytes in a skin equivalent model in vitro. Br. J. Dermatol. 119:503–512.
49. Gordon, P.R., Mansur, C.P., Gilchrest, B.A. (1989) Regulation of human melanocyte growth, dendricity, and melanization by keratinocyte derived factors. J. Invest. Dermatol. 92:565–572.
50. Coffey, R.J., Jr., Derynck, R., Wilcox, J.N., Bringman, T.S., Goustin, A.S., Moses, H.L., Pittelkow, M.R. (1987) Production and auto-induction of transforming growth factor-alpha in human keratinocytes. Nature 328:817–820.
51. Kupper, T.S., Chua, A.O., Flood, P., McGuire, J., Gubler, U. (1987) Interleukin 1 gene expression in cultured human keratinocytes is augmented by ultraviolet irradiation. J. Clin. Invest. 80:430–436.
52. Luger, T.A., Kock, A., Danner, M., Colot, M., Micksche, M. (1985) Production of distinct cytokines by epidermal cells. Br. J. Dermatol. 113(Suppl. 28):145–156.
53. Yaar, M., Palleroni, A.V., Gilchrest, B.A. (1986) Normal human epidermis contains an interferon-like protein. J. Cell. Biol. 103:1349–1354.
54. Torseth, J.W., Nickoloff, B.J., Basham, T.Y., Merigan, T.C. (1987) Beta interferon produced by keratinocytes in human cutaneous infection with herps simplex virus. J. Invest. Dis. 155:641–648.
55. Grossman, R.M., Krueger, J., Yourish, D., Granelli-Piperno, A., Murphy, D.P., May, L.T., Kupper, T.S., Schgal, P.B., Gottlieb, A.B. (1989) Interleukin-6 in expressed in high levels in psoriatic skin and stimulates proliferation of cultured human keratinocytes. Proc. Natl. Acad. Sci. USA 86:6367–6371.
56. Nickoloff, B.J. (1988) Keratinocytes produce a lymphocyte inhibitory factor which is

partially reversible by an antibody to transforming growth factor-beta. Ann. N.Y. Acad. Sci. 548:312–320.
57. Wikner, N.E., Persichitte, K.A., Baskin, J.B., Nielsen, L.D., Clark, R.A. (1988) Transforming growth factor-beta stimulates the expression of fibronection by human keratinocytes. J. Invest. Dermatol. 91:207–212.
58. Kupper, T.S., Lee, F., Goleman, D., Chodakewitz, J., Flood, D., Horowitz, M. (1988) Keratinocyte-derived T-cell growth factor is identical to granulocyte macrophage colony stimulating factor (GM-SCF). J. Invest. Dermatol. 91:185–188.

III

Metastases

6. Experimental model of human melanoma metastases

Dorothee Herlyn, Koji Adachi, Hilary Koprowski, and Meenhard Herlyn

1. Introduction

Models for spontaneous metastasis of human melanoma have recently been developed in nude mice [1–7]. These models have helped to define the three major steps within the metastatic cascade: cell attachment to basement membranes, membrane degradation, and cell locomotion [8]. Cells selected in these animal models have a relatively stable metastatic phenotype. Cultured cells from metastatic melanoma lesions, on the other hand, show instability of their metastatic phenotype. They are noninvasive when injected into nude mice [7] and have antigenic and genetic similarities with primary melanoma cells [9]. Instability of the metastatic properties of cells from metastatic lesions occurs either during in-vitro growth or as a result of variant selection during rapid proliferation in the human host [10].

We have developed a human melanoma metastasis model in nude mice. In this model, a human variant cell line (451-LU) was obtained that spontaneously metastasizes in nude mice. This variant cell line was selected from the lung of a nude mouse after several passages in vivo of human melanoma WM164 cells, which were previously isolated from a melanoma metastasis of a patient [11], but are without competence for metastasis in nude mice [7].

The phenotypes of the metastatic variant (451-LU) cells and nonmetastatic, parental (WM164) cells were compared with respect to growth at clonal cell densities, invasinveness of the cells, proteolytic enzyme activity, expression of melanoma-associated antigens, and karyotype. These studies demonstrate that metastatic cells, derived from a heterogeneous population of nonmetastatic cells, have distinct phenotypic characteristics, suggesting that metastases are produced by the selective growth of specialized aggressive subpopulations of metastatic cells that preexisted in the parent tumor, rather than by random survival of circulating tumor emboli.

This model has shown usefulness for the study of inhibition of human melanoma metastases by MAb in experimental animals. Although there are several reports on the inhibition of metastases of syngeneic animal tumors by antibodies [12–14], experimental models for the study of MAb effects on metastases of human tumors would provide useful information before the

L. Nathanson (ed.), MELANOMA RESEARCH: GENETICS, GROWTH FACTORS, METASTASES, AND ANTIGENS.

clinical application of MAb. MAb that inhibit the attachment of tumor cells to the basement membrane potentially may inhibit the metastatic spread of tumors invivo. Several melanoma-associated antigens have been implicated in the attachment of tumor cells to substrate, e.g., proteoglycan molecular complex (molecular masses of > 450 kD and 250 kD [15]) and chondroitin sulfate proteoglycan [16]. Gangliosides were shown, using MAbs, to localize in the focal adhesion plaques of tumor cells [17], and anti-ganglioside MAbs inhibited tumor growth in vitro in the absence of effector cells or complement [18]. In experimental animals, MAb to the GD_3 ganglioside suppressed subcutaneous growth of melanomas [19]. Clinical trials in melanoma patients indicate their possible usefulness of gangliosides as target antigens in passive immunotherapy [20].

We have shown [7] that MAb ME 36.1 to GD_2/GD_3 gangliosides inhibits experimental metastasis of human melanoma in nude mice. The availability of isotypic class switch variants of this MAb [21] greatly facilitated the analysis of the mechanism of metastasis inhibition by the anti-GD_2/GD_3 MAb.

2. Model of experimental spontaneous metastases of human melanoma

The procedures used to establish the model of spontaneous metastases of human melanoma in nude mice are schematized in Figure 1. Following i.v. injection of 1×10^6 WM164 cells into a nude mouse pretreated with β-estradiol to inactivate natural killer cells [22,23], a mass culture (first passage, 239-LU) was obtained from the lung. After confirming the human origin of the cultured cells by testing for binding with MAb to melanoma-associated antigens in mixed hemadsorption assay [9], 239-LU cells (1×10^6) were inoculated i.v. into five mice pretreated with β-estradiol. Human melanoma cells were cultured from the lungs of four mice. Cells (1×10^7) of one of the four cultures (282-LU, second passage) were inoculated s.c. into 4 β-estradiol-pretreated nude mice. Organs were excised after 6 weeks, and lung metastases that had formed spontaneously were cultured from two mice. Cells (1×10^7) of one culture (third passage, 417-LU) were inoculated s.c. into the flank of three mice not pretreated with β-estradiol. After 6 weeks, organs were excised again, and lung metastases were cultured from all three mice. Cells (5×10^6) of one culture (fourth passage, 451-LU mestastasis) were injected s.c. into four nude mice. All four mice showed grade III lung metastases 8 weeks after tumor cell inoculation (Figures 2a–2c). Single tumor cells (Figures 2d and 2e) were observed 2 weeks and 1 week after tumor cell inoculation, respectively. All mice also showed metastatic nodules in axillary lymph nodes. However, no metastases were found in any of the other organs tested, such as spleen, liver, and inguinal lymph nodes.

The characteristics of metastatic 451-LU in comparison to parental nonmetastatic WM164 cells are summarized in Table 1. We compared the phenotypes of the parental nonmetastatic cell line and of the metastatic

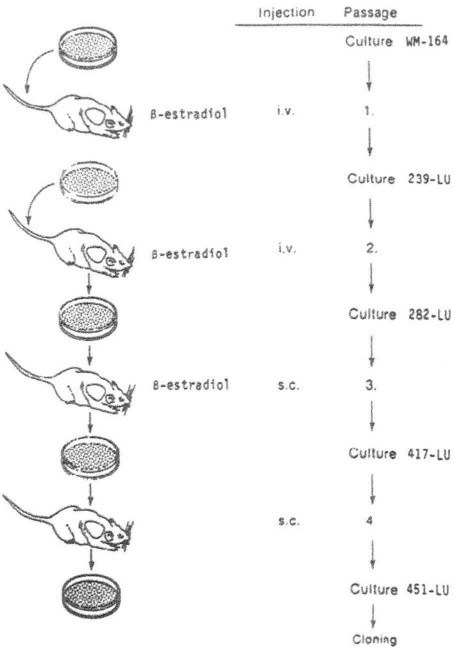

Figure 1. Isolation of metastatic variants of WM164 cells by sequential in-vivo/in-vitro passaging of the cells in nude mice and in culture. Mice were treated with β-estradiol implants [22] and tumor cells were injected either i.v. (1×10^6 cells) or s.c. (1×10^7 cells), followed by culturing of tumor cells from the lungs of nude mice after each injection.

variant with respect to growth behavior at clonal densities, in-vitro invasion through a reconstructed basement membrane, secretion of proteolytic enzymes, expression of tumor-associated antigens, and modal chromosome number. Metastatic 451-LU cells showed significantly increased growth rates [population doubling (PD) times], survival, and growth at clonal densities, as compared to the parental cell line. In an in-vitro invasion assay, metastatic 451-LU cells were shown to be significantly more invasive than the parental cells. The invasive variant secreted collagenase and tissue-type plasminogen activator (tPA) at levels ten- and threefold higher than those in the parental WM164 cells, respectively. In the metastatic cells, the percentage of cells expressing the NGF receptor was significantly increased. Furthermore, elevation of NGF receptor expression was also seen at the protein level (Western blot analysis) and transcriptional level (Northern blot analysis). The results obtained in indirect flow cytometry with MAb ME 36.1 against GD_2/GD_3 gangliosides indicate a greater than twofold increase in the percentage of cells binding MAb and a 1.8-fold increase in the mean fluorescence intensity per cell in 451-LU cells, as compared to WM164 cells. However, none of the other antigens tested, such as chondroitin sulfate proteoglycan

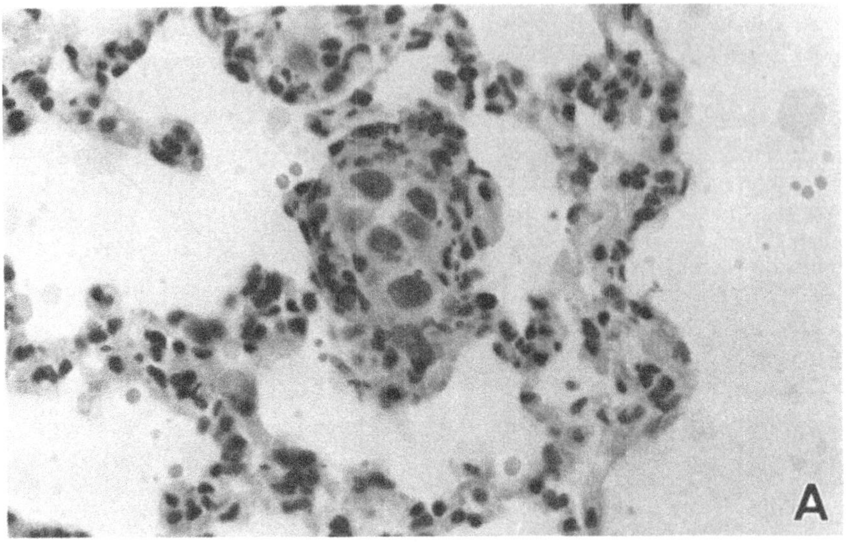

Figure 2. Metastases of 451-LU cells to the lungs of nude mice. A. Eight weeks after tumor cell inoculation, a small focus of tumor is seen within the lung parenchyma that is compatible with the establishment of a metastatic focus and does not represent simply cells floating loosely within the alveolar air space. Hematoxylin and eosin (magnification × 325).

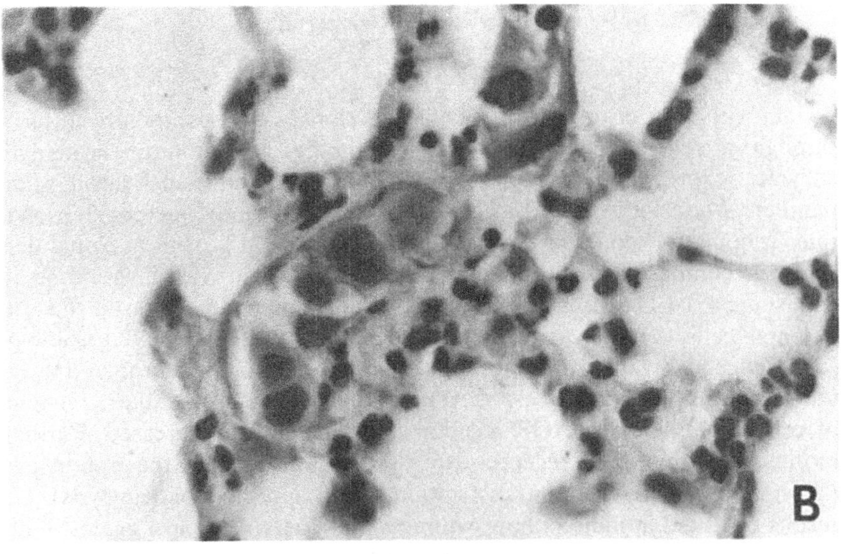

Figure 2. B. Several malignant cells are seen within a vessel in the lung parenchyma 8 weeks after tumor cell inoculation. Note the lining up of the malignant cells that are surrounded by flattened attenuated endothelium. This channel could be either a lymphatic or blood vessel. Hematoxylin and eosin (magnification × 650).

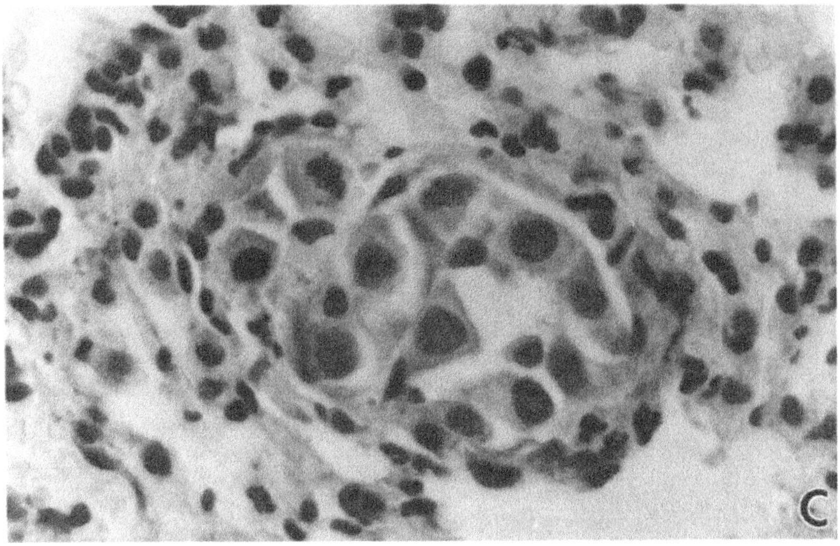

Figure 2. C. A grade III (> 10 cells per focus) metastatic tumor focus is seen within the lung parenchyma 8 weeks after tumor cell inoculation. The tumor cells are characterized by an increased size, increased nuclear-cytoplasmic ratio, and hyperchromatic nuclei with prominent nucleoli. Note the mitotic cell in the upper left-hand corner of the metastatic focus. Hematoxylin and eosin (magnification × 650).

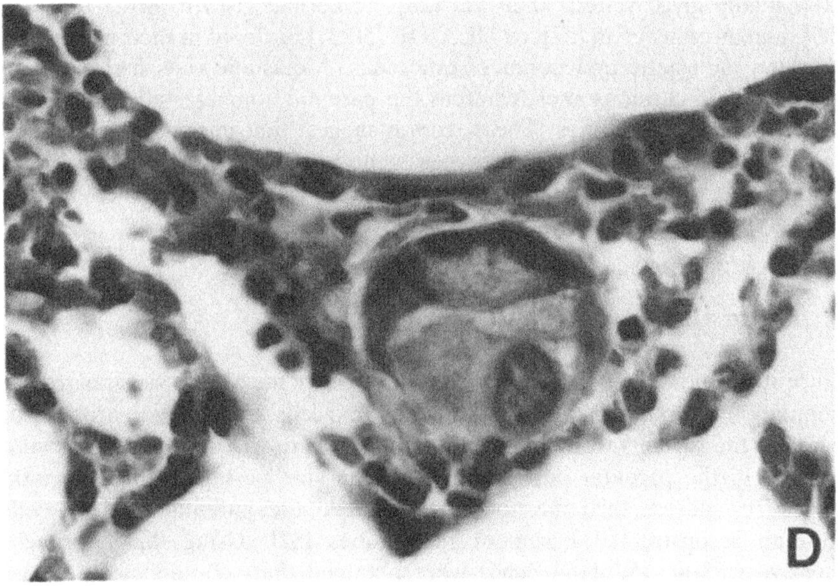

Figure 2. D. A single tumor cell is seen within the lung parenchyma 2 weeks after tumor cell inoculation (magnification × 325).

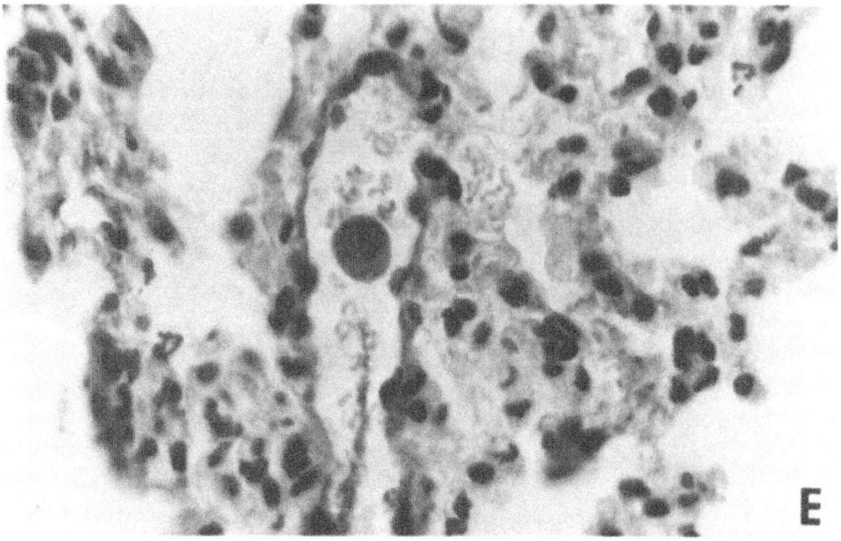

Figure 2. E. Isolated tumor cell within a blood vessel in the lung 7 days after tumor cell inoculation. Note the red blood cells within the channel. Hematoxylin and eosin (magnification × 650).

[24], proteins of 130/105 kD [25], 120 kD [25], 120/94 kD [26], 125/104/99 kD [27], highly glycosylated 30/60 kD [28], epidermal growth factor receptor [29], melanotransferrin [27], or HLA-DR [30,31], differed in their expression between metastatic and nonmetastatic cells. Metastatic cells had a modal number of 78 chromosomes, whereas the parental nonmetastatic cells had a mode of 52 chromosomes. These studies suggest that metastatic melanoma cell variants show distinct phenotypes, genotypes, and growth behavior, as compared to the nonmetastatic parental cells. The data further suggest phenotypic heterogeneity of the parental cells.

3. In-vitro selected invasive variants

Since it was possible to select in vivo in nude mice metastatic variants from a population of nonmetastatic human melanoma cells, the question arose as to whether the variants were 'induced' in nude mice or whether these cells were present in the parental population before in-vivo passaging through nude mice. To address this question, we passaged the parental WM164 cells through reconstructed basement membranes [32]. Using this approach, invasive variants (WM164-Bch4) were obtained that spontaneously metastasized in 100% of the nude mice. The in-vitro selected invasive cells showed characteristics similar to the in-vivo selected metastatic cells (Table 1). These

Table 1. Summary of characteristics of metastatic 451-LU and nonmetastatic WM164 melanoma cells

Parameter investigated	Parental cells WM164 (± S.D.)[a]	In-vivo selected metastatic cells 451-LU (± S.D.)[a]	In-vitro selected invasive cells WM164-Bch4 (± S.D.)[a]
Population doubling (PD) time (hr)[b]	222.1 ± 0.34	94 ± 16	166 ± 2.0
Colony-forming efficiency, CFE (%)[c]	2.0 ± 1.0	17 ± 5	14.0 ± 6.0
In-vitro invasiveness (number of cells migrated through Matrigel-covered filter in Boyden chamber)[d]	9.2 ± 3.1	25.6 ± 6.6	20.4 ± 0.0
Collagenase activity (ng/ml)[e]	0.05 ± 0.02	0.60 ± 0.25	n.t.
Tissue plasminogen activator (tPA) activity (mPU[f]/mg protein)[g]	8.5 ± 2.7	25.1 ± 9.5	16.4 ± 0.3
Percentage of cells expressing:			
NGF-receptor[h]	20 ± 5	100 ± 1.0	80 ± 10.0
GD_2/GD_3 gangliosides	10	28	n.t.
Chromosome mode[i]	52	78	90

[a] Mean ± S.D. (standard deviation) from two to three independently performed experiments.
[b] PD time was determined with cells grown in protein-free medium [49] and seeded at low densities (30–360 cells/cm^2) in wells precoated with 1% gelatin, and by counting cells at various days after seeding. PD time was calcualted as described [26].
[c] CFE was determined with cells grown at 180 cells/cm^2 as described under footnote (b) and CFE was calculated [26].
[d] Invasion of cells through a reconstructed basement membrane (Matrigel) was tested as described [32].
[e] Collagenase activity of cells grown in serum-free medium was determined in radioimmunoassay with ^{125}I-labeled type IV collagen as the substrate and bacterial collagenase type IV as the standard.
[f] mPU = milliploug unit.
[g] tPA activity was determined in supernatants of cells grown in serum-free medium by fibrin plate assay [50].
[h] Measured by mixed hemadsorption assay (NGF-receptor) [9] or FACS analysis (GD_2/GD_3).
[i] Determined by Giemsa banding of colchicine-treated cells [51].
The values shown for 451-LU and WM164-Bch 4 cells each differ significantly (at $p < 0.05$ level, Student's t test) from the corresponding values for WM164 cells for each parameter investigated.

results suggest that the parental nonmetastatic WM164 cells contained a subpopulation of cells that were invasive in vitro. It is hypothesized that these invasive cells gave rise to the in-vivo metastatic variants 451-LU.

4. Inhibition of experimental metastases by MAb ME 36.1

The model of experimental metastases of human melanoma described above served to test whether MAb ME 36.1 (IgG2a) defining the GD_2/GD_3 gangliosides [21] could inhibit metastatic spread of melanoma in nude mice. The

Table 2. Summary of inhibitory effects of MAb ME 36.1 on subcutaneous and metastatic growth of human melanoma cells[a]

MAb code	Day of administration after tumor cell inoculation[b]	Inhibition[c] of Primary (s.c. growing) tumor	Metastases (lung and axillary lymph node)
ME 36.1 (IgG2a)	0	yes[c]	yes[c]
	1	yes[c]	yes
	7	yes[c]	yes[c]
	14	no	no
ME 36.1 (IgG1)	0	no	yes[c]

[a] For details, see ref. 7.

[b] Nude mice were inoculated with 3×10^6 451-LU cells s.c. Following immediately (day 0) or at various time points (days 1, 7, 14) after tumor inoculation, mice were treated with 200 μg of MAb ME 36.1 or irrelevant control MAb i.p. daily for 2 weeks.

[c] Tumor sizes at the injection site and number of metastatic foci at distant organs were significantly (at $p < 0.05$ level, Student's t test) different in animals treated with MAb ME 36.1 as compared to animals treated with irrelevant control MAb.

results have been described in detail elsewhere [7] and are summarized in Table 2. When the MAb was injected on the day of tumor cell inoculation or 1 day thereafter, tumor growth at the injection site was completely inhibited, and no metastases were detected in popliteal lymph nodes or in the lungs, whereas mice treated with control antibody developed numerous metastases in those organs. Delayed MAb administration, i.e., 1 week after tumor inoculation, at a time when tumor cells had already metastasized to lymph nodes and lung, with MAb ME 36.1 significantly reduced the number of lung metastases. However, when the MAb was first administered 14 days after tumor inoculation, neither s.c. nor metastatic tumor growth were affected. Treatment of mice with an IgG1 variant immunoglobulin of MAb ME 36.1 [21] also resulted in significant inhibition of lung metastases formation but no inhibition of tumor growth at the primary site.

To clarify the mechanism of tumor growth inhibition by MAb ME 36.1 in nude mice, cytotoxic effects of the MAb in conjunction with effector cells or complement and the capacity of the MAb to inhibit cell invasion or attachment in vitro were investigated. MAb ME 36.1 of IgG2a isotype significantly lysed WM164 cells with human monocytes or lymphocytes as effector cells and serum as a source of complement [21]. MAb ME 36.1 of both isotypes (IgG1, IgG2a) inhibited cell attachment to substrate (Figure 3) as well as the invasion of cells through a reconstructed basement membrane (Matrigel) in vitro (Figure 4), whereas MAb ME 37.7 and ME 31.3 binding to HLA-DR and proteoglycan on melanoma cells, respectively, did not show significant inhibitory effects in these assays.

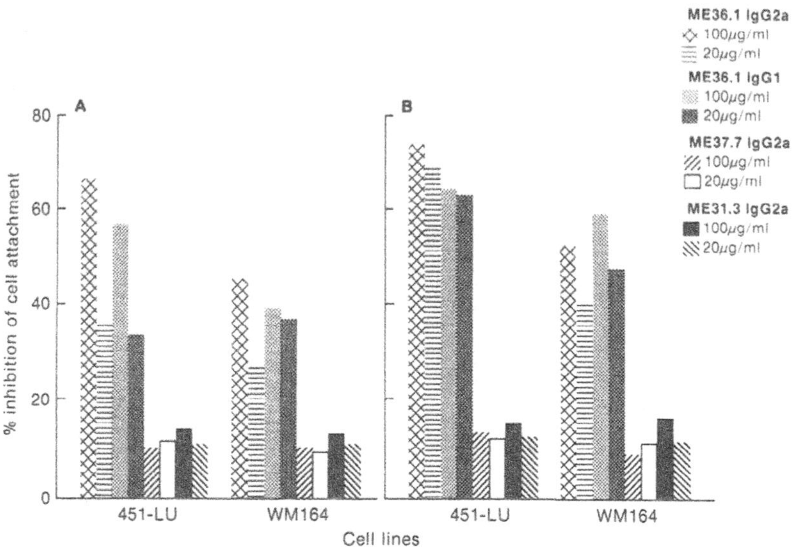

Figure 3. Inhibition of attachment of 451-LU and WM164 cells to gelatin-coated plastic plates by MAb ME 36.1 (IgG2a or IgG1, anti-GD_2/GD_3) and absence of inhibition by MAb ME 37.7 (IgG2a, anti-HLA-DR) and ME 31.3 (IgG2a, anti-proteoglycan). Cells grown in protein-free medium [49] were seeded into gelatin-coated wells after preincubating the cells with the various MAbs. Numbers of attached cells were determined as A: 45 minutes; B: 5 hours after plating. Inhibition was quantitated as the difference between the number of cells attached with and without preincubation with MAb and was expressed as the percentage of inhibition.

5. Conclusions

Melanoma cells, isolated from a metastatic lesion of a patient and maintained in culture, were shown to represent a heterogeneous population of cells with respect to metastatic capabilities in nude mice and invasiveness through a reconstructed basement membrane in vitro. Less than 1% of the parental WM164 cells spontaneously metastasized to the lungs of nude mice or invaded through a reconstructed membrane in vitro. Given the origin of WM164 from a melanoma metastasis of a patient, the fraction of metastatic/invasive cells seems rather low and is in the range of that reported for murine tumors [33]. Successful isolation from nonmetastatic WM164 cells of invasive variants in vitro, with metastatic properties in vivo (WM164-Bch4 cells), suggests that a subpopulation of invasive cells present a priori in the parental nonmetastatic cells gave rise to the metastatic 451-LU cell line that was isolated under selective pressure in vivo. This is further supported by the similarities in phenotypic differences observed in the in-vitro and in-vivo selected variants when compared to the nonmetastatic parent line. Phenotypic differences between metastatic/invasive and the parental cells were found with respect to invasiveness, proteolytic enzymes, expression of

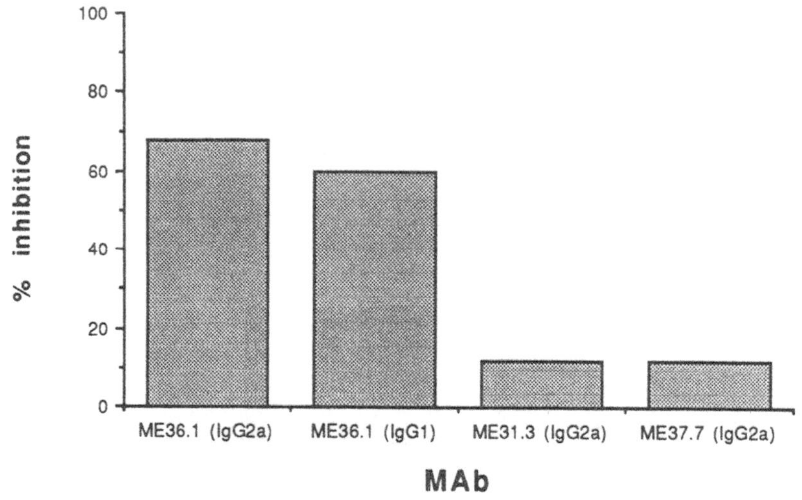

Figure 4. Inhibition of cell invasion by MAb ME 36.1 (IgG2a or IgG1, anti-GD_2/GD_3), absence of inhibition by MAb ME 31.3 (IgG2a, anti-proteoglycan) and ME 37.7 (IgG2a, anti-HLA-DR). Cell invasion through a reconstructed membrane in a Boyden chamber was measured as described [7].

melanoma-associated antigens, and karyotype. The demonstration of distinct phenotypic differences between metastatic/invasive and nonmetastatic cells seems to indicate that metastases are produced by the selective growth of specialized aggressive subpopulations of cells that preexisted in the parent tumor, rather than by random survival of circulating tumor emboli [34,35].

A striking difference between nonmetastatic and metastatic/invasive melanoma cells is the increased growth factor independence at low cell density of the latter cells. Similar results have been recently reported by others for human melanoma cells [36] and murine tumor cells [37–39]. Independence from exogeneous growth factors and higher survival at clonal (nonoptimal) cell densities may be due to the production of growth factors for autocrine growth stimulation, several of which have recently been demonstrated in melanoma cells, including transforming growth factor alpha [40], platelet-derived growth factor [41], and fibroblast growth factor [42].

The increase in the invasiveness of melanoma cell variants as compared to the parental cells might be at least partially explained by the increased tPA and collagenolytic activity in the variant cells. Invasiveness was significantly inhibited by preincubation of the cells with antibodies to tPA.

We have demonstrated here that metastatic 451-LU cells have increased the expression of GD_2/GD_3 gangliosides and NGF-receptor protein and mRNA. Whereas the role of the NGF receptor in metastasis is highly speculative, gangliosides have been implicated in the attachment of tumor cells to substrate [17], and the increased ganglioside level in 451-LU cells may relate to the invasiveness of these cells.

Both variants of WM164 cells showed extra chromosomes 7 and 20. While the role of chromosome 20 in tumor progression is unclear, interesting associations have been found with respect to chromosome 7. It seems that genes involved in invasion and metastasis are located on human chromosome 7 [43]. Extra chromosome 7 has been detected in advanced metastatic melanomas and has been shown to be associated with high expression of the epidermal growth factor receptor [44].

This model of spontaneous metastasis to regional lymph nodes and lungs after s.c. injection of melanoma cells into nude mice mimics closely the metastatic route of melanoma in patients. The model has been useful for the study of metastasis inhibition by MAb. MAb ME 36.1 to GD_2/GD_3 gangliosides was chosen for these studies because gangliosides most likely are involved in the metastatic spread of melanoma [17,18]. IgG2a MAb ME 36.1 significantly inhibited tumor growth at the inoculation site as well as metastatic spread to lymph nodes and lungs. On the other hand, IgG1 MAb ME 36.1 did not significantly inhibit tumor growth at the injection site but significantly inhibited metastatic spread of tumor cells. Inhibition of melanoma growth at the injection site by IgG2a MAb ME 36.1 might be mediated primarily by macrophages (as shown for other IgG2a MAbs against human tumors [45]), since the MAb is highly cytotoxic against cultured melanoma cells in conjunction with murine or human macrophages/monocytes.

The exact mechanism by which metastatic spread of melanoma cells is inhibited by both the IgG2a and IgG1 MAb ME 36.1 is not known. On the basis of our data obtained in vitro (Figures 3 and 4), we speculate that inhibition of cell attachment to endothelial cell and/or basement membranes and/or inhibition of invasion may have played a role in vivo. Alternative mechanisms of inhibition of metastasis by MAb ME 36.1 include clearance of MAb-coated tumor cells from the circulation, either by cells of the reticuloendothelial system or complement. In animal tumor models, inhibition of metastases by antibodies directed to various tumor-associated antigens has been attributed to the clearance of antibody-coated cells from the vasculation by effector cells and/or complement [14,46,47].

MAb ME 36.1 clearly showed immunotherapeutic potential in the nude mouse model. The first clinical trial with this MAb in 13 melanoma patients has shown encouraging results [48]. One patient with multiple skin lesions showed a complete response and has been free of detectable disease for more than 2 years as of 1990.

Acknowledgments

We thank Shirley Peterson for excellent editorial assistance. This study was support by National Institutes of Health grants CA25874, CA10815, and CA6027001.

References

1. Kerbel, R.S., Man, M.S., Dexter, D. (1984) A model of human cancer metastasis: Extensive spontaneous and artificial metastasis of a human pigmented melanoma and derived variant sublines in nude mice. J. Natl. Cancer Inst. 72:93–108.
2. Kozlowski, J.M. Fidler, I.J., Campbell, D., Xu, Z.L., Kaighn, M.E., Hart, I.R. (1984) Metastatic behavior of human tumor cell line growth in the nude mouse. Cancer Res. 44:3522–3529.
3. Gitelman, I., Dexter, D.F., Roder, J.C. (1987) DNA amplification and metastasis of the human melanoma cell line MeWo. Cancer Res. 47:3851–3855.
4. Zimmerman, R.J., Gaillard, E.T., Goldin, A. (1987) Metastatic potential of four human melanoma xenografts in young athymic mice following tail vein inoculation. Cancer Res. 47:2305–2310.
5. Ishikawa, M., Fernandez, B., Kerbel, R.S. (1988) Highly pigmented human melanoma variant which metastasizes widely in nude mice, including to skin and brain. Cancer Res. 48:4897–4903.
6. Fodstad, O., Kjonniksen, I., Aamdal, S. (1988) Extrapulmonary, tissue-specific metastasis formation in nude mice injected with FEMX-1 human melanoma cells. Cancer Res. 48:4382–4388.
7. Iliopoulos, D., Ernst, C., Stwplewski, Z., Jambrosic, J., Rodeck, U., Herlyn, M., Clark, W.H. Jr., Koprowski, H., Herlyn, D. (1989) Inhibition of metastases of a human melanoma xenograft by monoclonal anitybody to the GD_2/GD_3 gangliosides. J. Natl. Cancer Inst. 81:440–444.
8. Liotta, L.A. (1986) Tumor invasion and metastases. Role of the extracellular matrix. Cancer Res. 46:1–7.
9. Herlyn, M., Balaban, G., Bennicelli, J., Guery, D., IV, Halaban, R., Herlyn, D., Elder, D.E., Maul, G.G., Steplewski, Z., Nowell, P.C., Clark, W.H., Koprowski, H. (1985) Primary melanoma cells of the vertical growth phase: Similarities to metastatic cells. J. Natl. Cancer Inst. 74:283–289.
10. Kerbel, R.S., Waghorne, C., Korczak, B., Lagarde, A., Breitman, M. (1988) Clonal dominance of primary tumours by metastatic cells: Genetic analysis and biological implications. Cancer Surveys 7:597–629.
11. Herlyn, M., Clark, W.H. Jr., Mastrangelo, M.J., Guerry, D. IV, Elder, D.E., LaRossa, D., Hamilton, R., Bondi, E., Tuthill, R., Steplewski, Z., Koprowski, H. (1980) Specific immunoreactivity of monoclonal antimelanoma antibodies. Cancer Res. 40:3602–3609.
12. Vollmers, H.P., Birchmeier, W. (1983) Monoclonal antibodies inhibit the adhesion of mouse B16 melanoma cells in vitro and black lung metastasis in vivo. Proc. Natl. Acad. Sci. USA 80:3729–3733.
13. Ukei, S., Saiki, I., Azuma, I. (1985) Monoclonal antibodies to Lewis lung carcinoma. J. Cancer Res. Clin. Oncol. 110:103–109.
14. Gunji, Y., Taniguchi, M. (1986) Syngeneic monoclonal antimelanoma antibody that inhibits experimental lung metastasis of B16 melanoma. Jpn. J. Cancer Res. 77:595–601.
15. deVries, J.E., Keizer, G.D., teVelde, A.A., Voordauw, A., Ruiter, P., Spits, H., Figdor, C.G. (1986) Characterization of melanoma-associated surface antigens invovled in the adhesion and motility of human melanoma cells. Int. J. Cancer 38:465–473.
16. Bumol, T.F., Reisfeld, R.A. (1982) Unique glycoprotein-proteoglycan complex defined by monoclonal antibody on human melanoma cells. Proc. Natl. Acad. Sci. USA 79:1245–1249.
17. Cheresh, P.A., Harper, J.R., Schulz, G., Reisfeld, R.A. (1984) Localization of the gangliosides GD_2 and GD_3 in adhesion plaques and on the surface of human melanoma cells. Proc. Natl. Acad. Sci. USA 81:5767–5771.
18. Dippold, W.G., Knuth, A., zum Buschenfelde, K.-H. (1984) Inhibition of human melanoma cell growth in vitro by monoclonal anti-GD_3-ganglioside antibody. Cancer Res. 44:806–810.
19. Cheresh, D.A., Hansik, C.J., Staffileno, L.K., Jung, G., Reisfeld, R.A. (1985) Disialo-

ganglioside GD_3 on human melanoma serves as a relevant target for monoclonal antibody-mediated tumor cytolysis. Proc. Natl. Acad. Sci. USA 82:5155–5159.

20. Houghton, A.N., Mintzer, D., Cordon-Cardo, C., Welt, S., Fliegel, B., Vadhan, S., Carswell, E., Melamed, M.R., Oettgen, H.F., Old, L.J. (1985) Mouse monoclonal IgG3 antibody detecting GD3 ganglioside: A phase I trial in patients with malignant melanoma. Proc. Natl. Acad. Sci. USA 82:1242–1246.
21. Thurin, J., Thurin, M., Kimoto, Y., Herlyn, M., Lubeck, M.D., Elder, D.E., Smereczynska, M., Karlsson, K.A., Clark, W.H. Jr., Steplewski, Z., Koprowski, H. (1987) Monoclonal antibody-defined correlation in melanoma between levels of GD_2 and GD_3 antigens and antibody-mediated cytotoxicity. Cancer Res. 47:1229–1233.
22. Hanna, N., Schneider, M. (1983) Enhancement of tumor metastasis and suppression of natural killer cell activity by β-estradiol treatment. J. Immunol. 130:974–980.
23. Sharkey, F.E., Fogh, J. (1979) Metastasis of human tumors in athymic nude mice. Int. J. Cancer 24:733–742.
24. Ross, A.H., Herlyn, M. Ernst, C.S., Guerry, D., Bennicelli, J., Ghrist, B.F.D., Atkinson, B., Koprowski, H. (1984) Immunoassay for melanoma-associated proteoglycan in sera of patients using monoclonal and polyclonal antibodies. Cancer Res. 44:4642–4647.
25. Herlyn, M., Thurin, J., Balaban, G., Bennicelli, J.L., Herlyn, D., Elder, D.E., Bondi, E., Guerry, D., Nowell, P.C., Clark, W.H., Koprowski, H. (1985) Characteristics of cultured human melanocytes isolated from different stages of tumor progression. Cancer Res. 45:5670–5676.
26. Herlyn, M., Rodeck, U., Mancianti, M.L., Cardillo, F.M., Lang, A., Ross, A.H., Jambrosic, J., Koprowski, H. (1987) Expression of melanoma-associated antigens in cultured rapidly dividing human melanocytes. Cancer Res. 47:3057–3061.
27. Herlyn, M., Steplewski, Z., Herlyn, D., Clark, W.H., Ross, A.H., Blaszczyk, M., Pak, K.Y., Koprowski, H. (1983) Production and characterization of monoclonal antibodies against human malignant melanoma. Cancer Invest. 1:215–224.
28. Atkinson, B., Ernst, C.S., Ghrist, B.F.D., Ross, A.H., Clark, W.H., Herlyn, M., Herlyn, D., Maul, G.G., Steplewski, Z., Koprowski, H. (1985) Monoclonal antibody to a highly glycosylated protein reacts in fixed tissue with melanoma and other tumors. Hybridoma 4:243–255.
29. Rodeck, U., Herlyn, M., Herlyn, D., Molthoff, C., Atkinson, B., Vorello, M., Steplewski, Z., Koprowski, H. (1987) Tumor growth inhibition by a monoclonal antibody to the epidermal growth factor receptor: Immunologically mediated and effector cell independent effects. Cancer Res. 47:3692–3696.
30. Koprowski, H., Steplewski, Z., Herlyn, D., Herlyn, M. (1978) Study of antibodies against human melanoma produced by somatic cell hybrids. Proc. Natl. Acad. Sci. USA 75:3405–3409.
31. Lloyd, K.O., Ng, J., Dippold, W.G. (1981) Analysis of the biosynthesis of HLA-DR glycoproteins in human malignant melanoma cell lines. J. Immunol. 126:2408–2413.
32. Albini, A., Iwamoto, Y., Kleinman, H.U., Martin, G.R., Aaronson, S.A., Kozlowski, J.M., McEwan, R.N. (1987) A rapid in vitro assay for quantitating invasive potential of tumor cells. Cancer Res. 47:3239–3245.
33. Fidler, I.J., Talmadge, J.E. (1986) Evidence that intravenously derived murine pulmonary melanoma metastases can originate from the expansion of a single tumor cell. Cancer Res. 46:5167–5171.
34. Talmadge, J.E., Fidler, I.J. (1982) Cancer metastasis is selective or random depending on the parent tumor population. Nature (London) 297:593–597.
35. Talmadge, J.E., Fidler, I.J. (1982) Enhanced metastatic potential of tumor cells harvested from spontaneous metastases of heterogeneous murine tumor. J. Nat. Cancer Inst. 69:975–980.
36. Sauvaigo, S., Fretts, R.E., Riopelle, R.J., Lagarde, A.E. (1986) Autonomous proliferation of MeWo human melanoma cell lines in serum-free medium: Secretion of growth-stimulating activities. Int. J. Cancer 37:123–132.

37. Chadwick, D.E., Lagarde, A.E. (1988) Coincidental acquisition of growth autonomy and metastatic potential during malignant transformation of factor-dependent CCL39 lung fibroblasts. J. Natl. Cancer Inst. 80:318–325.
38. Ethier, S.P., Cundiff, K.C. (1987) Importance of extended growth potential and growth factor independence on in vivo neoplastic potential of primary rat mammary carcinoma cells. Cancer Res. 47:5316–5322.
39. Waghorne, C., Thomas, M., Lagarde, A., Kerbel, R.S., Breitman, M.L. (1988) Genetic evidence for progressive selection and overgrowth of primary tumors by metastatic cell subpopulations. Cancer Res. 48:6109–6114.
40. Richmond, A., Lawson, D.H., Nixon, D.W., Stevens, J.S., Chawla, R.K. (1983) Extraction of a melanoma growth-stimulatory activity from culture medium conditioned by the HS0294 human melanoma cell line. Cancer Res. 43:2106–2112.
41. Westermark, B., Johnsson, A., Paulsson, Y., Betscholtz, C., Heldin, C.-H., Herlyn, M., Rodeck, U., Koprowski, H. (1986) Human melanoma cell lines of primary and metastatic origin express the genes encoding the chains of platelet-derived growth factor (PDGF) and produce a PDGF-like growth factor. Proc. Natl. Acad. Sci. USA 83:7197–7200.
42. Moscatelli, D., Presta, M., Joseph-Silverstein, J., Rifkin, D.B. (1986) Both normal and tumor cells produce basic fibroblast growth factor. J. Cell Physiol. 129:273–276.
43. Collard, J.G., VanDePoll, M., Scheffer, A., Ross, E., Hopman, A.H.M., Geurts van Kessel, A.H.M., van Dongen, J.J.M. (1987) Location of genes involved in invasion and metastasis on human chromosome 7. Cancer Res. 47:6666–6670.
44. Koprowski, H., Herlyn, M., Balaban, G., Parmiter, A., Ross, A.H., Nowell, P.C. (1985) Expression of the receptor for epidermal growth factor correlates with increased dosage of chromosome 7 in malignant melanoma. Somat. Cell Mol. Genet. 11:297–301.
45. Herlyn, D., Koprowski, H. (1982) IgG2a monoclonal antibodies inhibit human tumor growth through interaction with effector cells. Proc. Natl. Acad. Sci. USA 79:4761–4765.
46. Stavrou, D., Mellert, W., Mellert, U., Keiditsch, E., Bise, K., Mehraein, P. (1986) Growth inhibition of experimental glioma grafts by monoclonal antibody treatment. J. Cancer Res. Clin. Oncol. 112:111–118.
47. Badger, C.C., Bernstein, I.D. (1983) Therapy of murine leukemia with monoclonal antibody against a normal differentiation antigen. J. Exp. Med. 157:828–842.
48. Lichtin, A., Iliopoulós, D., Guerry, D., Elder, D., Herlyn, D., Steplewski, Z. (1988) Therapy of melanoma with an anti-melanoma ganglioside monoclonal antibody: A possible mechansim of a complete response. Proc. Am. Soc. Clin. Oncol. 7:247.
49. Rodeck, U., Herlyn, M., Menssen, H.D., Furlanetto, R.W., Koprowski, H. (1987) Metastatic but not primary melanoma cell lines grow in vitro independently of exogenous growth factors. Int. J. Cancer 40:687–690.
50. Morioka, S., Lazarus, G.S., Jensen, P.J. (1987) Involvement of urokinase type plasminogen activator in acantholysis induced by pemphigus IgG. J. Invest. Dermatol. 89:474–477.
51. Balaban, G., Herlyn, M., Guerry, D. IV, Bartolo, R., Koprowski, H., Clark, W.H., Nowell, P.C. (1984) Cytogenetics of human malignant melanoma and premalignant lesions. Cancer Genet. Cytogenet. 11:429–439.

7. The role of metalloproteinases in tumor cell metastasis

Richard M. Schultz

1. Introduction

Metastasis is a complex process for which the controlling factors have not yet been clearly identified. While certain oncogene transformations of cells will generate a metastatic phenotype, other transformations by even the same oncogene lead to cells having an ability to form a tumor but lacking an ability to metastasize [1]. It is thus unclear whether the generation of the metastatic phenotype is a genetic or an epigenetic event. It may be an inducible phenotype of a transformed cell, due to factors in the environment of the cell. Different cellular phenotypes may be induced during the different steps in metastases: detachment from a primary tumor, invasion through the basement membranes surrounding tissues and intravasation into the blood or lymph vasculature, survival from any immunological assault, adherence to the vascular wall of its target organ, extravasation from the vasculature, and proliferation at its new site. A critical part of the process is the invasion through the connective tissue stroma and basement membranes that surround organs and tissues, including the blood and lymph systems. Metalloproteinases secreted by tumor cells or by nontransformed cells associated with the tumor cells are believed to facilitate the process. This chapter will review aspects of the role of these metalloproteinases and their inhibitors in the metastatic process. The reader may also wish to consult other recent reviews on this subject [2,3].

2. Metalloproteinase structure

Three distinct metalloproteinase activities have been correlated with the metastatic phenotype of transformed cells: type I collagenase (matrix metalloproteinase 1, MMP-1), type IV collagenase (matrix metalloproteinase 2, MMP-2), and stromelysin (matrix metalloproteinase 3, MMP-3). These enzymes are synthesized and secreted as proenzyme forms, which must be activated extracellularly by specific proteolysis. Two distinct genetic forms of type IV procollagenases with molecular weights 72 kD and 92 kD have been identified in the human. The cDNA sequences for both forms have been

L. Nathanson (ed.), MELANOMA RESEARCH: GENETICS, GROWTH FACTORS, METASTASES, AND ANTIGENS.

determined [4,5]. Type I procollagenase has been isolated in a variety of cell types, and the human type I procollagenase has been cloned [6]. It is found in minor amounts as a glycoprotein with a mass of 57 kD and in its major form as a unglycosylated protein with a mass of 52 kD. Stromelysin has been purified, sequenced, and cloned [7]. It is also secreted in two forms, a 57-kD form, and in minor amounts as a glycosylated 60 kD protein [8]. More than one stromelysin gene has been isolated [9]. The metalloproteinase transin isolated and cloned from rodent cells has been shown to be homologous to human stromelysin [7,8]. A metallohydrolase with endoglycosidase activity is reportedly present in higher concentrations in the culture media of more metastatic murine B16 melanoma cells [10]. This activity may be due to stromelysin (MMP-3) [11].

A new collagenolytic protease, pump-1, has been recently isolated by screening a human tumor cDNA library with a rat stromelysin probe under low stringency [12]. Pump-1 is synthesized as a proenzyme of molecular weight 28,000, and is processed to yield active species of molecular weights 21,000 and 19,000.

The human prometalloproteinases possess an overall structural homology [4]. The amino acid sequence alignment shows that prostromelysin and type I procollagenase are more closely related to each other than to type IV procollagenase (72-kD form). A similar NH_2-terminal domain (192 residues in type IV procollagenase) is conserved in all three proteases. The COOH-terminal domain (264 residues in type IV collagenase) also appears to be homologous in all three metalloproteinases. The central domain of type IV procollagenase is not homologous with type I procollagenase of prostromelysin, and consists of a 58-residue motif repeated three times in tandem. This unique motif is positioned directly in front of the conserved sequence of the putative zinc binding site, which is probably the catalytic site of the enzyme. These type IV procollagenase repeats have a homology to the collagen binding domain in fibronectin. The 92-kD procollagenase consists of five domains: the NH_2-terminal and COOH-terminal domains present in all metalloproteinases, a zinc binding domain, and the fibronectin-like collagen binding domain that is also present in the 72-kD type IV collagenase. In addition, the 92-kD type IV collagenase contains a 54-amino acid long proline-rich domain homologous to the sequence in the *alpha*(2) chain of type V collagen. Pump-1 has a sequence homology to stromelysin and type I collagenase, but lacks the COOH-terminal domain characteristic of these enzymes [12]. The procollagenases are activated by a proteolytic cleavage, which removes approximately 80 amino acids from their NH_2-terminal end [4–8,12].

3. Substrate specificity of the metalloproteinases

It has been generally found that type IV collagenase cleaves types IV and V collagens and not interstitial collagens types I–III. In turn, type I collagenase is active against interstitial collagens, and not type IV and V collagens. However, the substrate specificities of the three metalloproteinases overlap to some extent, depending on the source and prior treatment of the substrate. Collier et al. [4] have studied the substrate specificity of the three human matrix metalloproteinases. Type IV collagenase is the same enzyme that was previously designated gelatinase, and it has a high activity against denatured type I collagen (gelatin). However, only type I collagenase acts on type I collagen in its folded triple-helical conformation. Stromelysin has a similar activity as type IV collagenase to type IV collagen secreted from the Engelbreth-Holm-Swarm (EHS) tumor, and even type I collagenase has a low activity towards EHS type IV collagen. However, only type IV collagenase had a detectable activity towards placental type IV collagen. All three matrix metalloproteinases have fibronectin degradative activities, but only stromelysin was observed to act on laminin. In addition, stromelysin degrades proteoglycans and fibronectin [5,13]. The substrate specificity of the 92-kD type IV procollagenase appears indistinguishable from that of the 72-kD type IV collagenase [4]. Pump-1 hydrolyzes gelatins (denatured forms) of types I, III, IV, and V collagen, and fibronectin, and can activate type I procollagenase [12].

4. Structure and composition of the extracellular matrix

A significant part of the volume of tissues is the extracellular space, occupied by a complex network of macromolecules which comprise the extracellular matrix. The extracellular matrix includes the basement membranes and the connective tissue stromas. The basement membrane or *basal lamina* is an extremely thin but tough membrane that separates tissues of different immunological types. A continuous basement membrane surrounds the vessels of the lymph and blood systems through which tumor cells metastasize. The basement membrane consists of heparin sulfate proteoglycans, type IV collagen, laminin, entactin, and other glycoproteins. The connective tissue stroma beneath the basement membrane is composed of interstitial collagen types I, II, and III, fibronectin, elastin, proteoglycans, hyaluronic acid, and other glyocoproteins.

Type IV collagen thus provides the molecular framework for the basement membrane. These collagen molecules do not form extracellular fibrils, as found for interstitial collagens (types I–III), but apparently polymerize in a defined polygonal network structure that forms an extended sheet-like lattice [14]. Laminar lattices in different planes are interconnected by disulfide cross-links between the collagen molecules. Type V collagen is found in basement membrane near its interface with the interstitial stroma.

In addition to type IV collagen, laminin is a major protein constituent of the basement membrane. Laminin is a large protein (~850,000 Dal) composed of three polypeptide chains, which electron microscopy shows to be arranged in the shape of a cross, held together at their intersection by disulfide bonds [15]. The two short arms of the cross are determined by each of the two smaller polypeptide chains B1 and B2, each about 200 kD, while the long part of the cross-like structure is primarily due to the larger 400-kD A polypeptide chain. The structure contains multiple functional domains. One of the domains in laminin has a binding site for type IV collagen, a second binds to the heparin sulfate of basement membrane, and a third domain binds to the surface of cells through laminin receptors. The cell-binding domain of the laminin molecule contains the amino acid sequence YIGSR (tyrosine-isoleucine-glycine-serine-arginine), which is essential to the cell-binding property of laminin. The concentration of cell-surface YIGSR binding laminin receptors has been correlated with metastatic potential [16]. It has been shown that treatment of murine B16 melanoma cells with the YIGSR pentapeptide prior to their injection in C57BL mice will significantly inhibit their ability to colonize the mouse lung [17]. These experiments show the importance of laminin receptors in the extravasation step of the metastatic process.

Fibronectin is an adhesive glycoprotein of the stroma, like laminin in basement membrane [18]. Fibronectin molecules are also composed of multiple domains that have binding sites for collagen, heparin, fibrin, and cell surface receptors. The fibronectin molecules are dimers of two polypeptide chains joined by disulfide bonds near their COOH-terminal ends. Each of the two distinct chains are very large, with approximately 2500 amino acids per polypeptide chain. In the extracellular matrix and on the cell surface, fibronectin molecules are further cross-linked to one another by additional disulfide bonds and often form insoluble fibronectin fibrils through the stroma. The amino acids in its cell-binding domain responsible for the binding of fibrin to cells contain the sequence RGDS (arginine-glycine-aspartate-serine). Other glycoproteins of the extracellular matrix also contain this sequence, and these adhesive extracellular matrix proteins bind to specific RGD cell receptors known as integrins [19]. Similar to the case of the laminin YIGSR sequence, treatment of B16 murine melanoma cells with the RGDS sequence prevents cells from strongly adhering to extracellular matrix and inhibits lung colonization following injection into C57BL mice [20].

5. Mechanism of extracellular matrix invastion

Liotta [2] has proposed a mechanism of tumor cell invasion through basement membrane of the extracellular matrix. In this mechanism the tumor cell first attaches to the laminin of the basement membrane through its laminin receptors. The binding of laminin to the laminin receptors induce the cell to secrete collagenase type IV and other proteolytic enzymes, which degrade the extracellular matrix components in the region of the cell, generating a path for cell movement through the basement membrane. The cell transverses the membrane by repeating in a stepwise fashion the steps of attachment to laminin, secretion of hydrolytic degradative activity, followed by cell locomotion into the region of the proteolytically modified extracellular matrix. It is inferred that tumor cell migration through the connective tissue stroma would similarly involve stepwise attachments to fibronectin with secretion of degradative enzymes.

6. Evidence in support of the involvement of metalloproteinases in the stepwise mechanism of extracellular matrix invasion

6.1. Correlation of metalloproteinase activity with metastatic potential

There are multiple reports showing increases in the synthesis and/or secretion of metalloproteinases with transformation, metastatic potential, and on treatment with tumor promoters [2,3]. The evidence is particularly strong for type IV collagenase activity [2,3,21]. For example, a strong correlation was observed between metastatic potential in *ras*-oncogene transfected early passage rat embryo fibroblasts and type IV collagenase activity [22]. The c-Ha-*ras* oncogene alone, or combined with v-*myc*, induced these cells to secrete high levels of type IV collagenolytic activity and showed a correspondingly high incidence of spontaneous metastasis from primary tumors grown in nude mice. In contrast, the cotransfection of *ras* plus the adenovirus type 2 Ela gene gave cells that grew tumors but were not metastatic. These latter cells also failed to produce type IV collagenase. Similar results showing a correlation between metastatic ability and the secretion of type IV collagenolytic activity were obtained with oncogene transformations of NIH 3T3 cells [23]. In this case [23], the synthesis of the larger 92-kD type IV procollagenase was correlated with metastatic potential. The 92-kD procollagenase was reported to be secreted by SV40-transformed human lung fibroblasts, but not in the untransformed parental cell line IMR-90. However H-*ras* transformed human bronchial epithelial cells (TBE-1) were shown to secrete only the 72-kD type IV procollagenase [4].

While a correlation with type IV collagenase activity and metastatic ability has been established for many cell lines some contradictory reports exist [4,24,25]. Whether there is a strong positive correlation of a particular metalloproteinase with metastasis may depend on the cell type and the presence or absence of environmental stimulators.

Stromelysin and type I collagenase activities have also been sometimes correlated with metastatic potential [3,6,8]. Stromelysin/transin mRNA was shown to be increased in mouse skin carcinomas in comparison to normal skin or benign papaillomas [26, 27]. Increases in stromelysin were observed in transformed and metastatic Swiss 3T3 cells [28]. However, Collier et al. reported that human endothelial cells, keratinocytes, melanoma cells (A2508), fibrosarcoma cells (HT-1080), and SV40-transformed human fetal lung fibroblasts do not express stromelysin, nor is the enzyme induced by phorbol ester [4].

6.2. *The induction of collagenase activity by laminin and fibronectin*

Laminin at concentrations of 4–8 μg/ml added to the serum-free media of human melanoma A2058 cells increased the type IV collagenase activity two- to threefold [29]. An increase in type IV collagenase activity of sixfold was observed when laminin fragments, as opposed to whole laminin, was added to the culture media. The studies support the idea that tumor cell binding to laminin, which comprises the first step of the basement membrane invasion mechanism, will induce the second step, the collagenolytic destruction of the basement membrane in the vicinity of the tumor cell.

Fibronectin fragments, but not whole fibronectin, could induce type I collagenase and stromelysin gene expressions in cultured rabbit synovial fibroblasts [30]. Collagen fragments, perhaps produced by the degradative action of the metalloproteinases, have been shown to be chemotactic for some tumor cells [31].

6.3. *An inhibitor of metalloproteinases can inhibit metastasis*

Tissue inhibitor of metalloproteinases (TIMP), a small glycoprotein of molecular weight 28,500 Da, is synthesized by many, if not all, fetal and adult human tissues of mesodermal origin [32]. It is a stoichiometric inhibitor of all the metalloendoproteinases described, including the type I collagenases (interstitial collagenases), the type IV collagenases, the stromelysins, and the pump-1 protease [3,12,33–46]. Immunologically identical forms of TIMP are detected in a wide variety of human body fluids [37]. While it is present in serum, its function in serum is not clear. Alpha-2 macroglobulin is also a collagenase inhibitor and provides the bulk of the anti-collagenase activity of serum [37,38]. TIMP has been found in high concentration in platelets and is presumably secreted into blood on platelet activation [39]. The protein has been isolated [40], sequenced [40–43], and cloned by several groups [41–43]. It is identical to a protein reported to have erythroid potentiating activity (EPA) [41,42]. The TIMP gene has been assigned to the X chromosome [44].

As TIMP is an important physiological inhibitor of metalloproteinases, it may have a significant role in modulating the invasion of tumor cells through extracellular matrix. In in-vitro experiments using the amniotic membrane from the human placenta to model invasion of tumor cells across basement membrane and collagenous stroma, low concentrations of TIMP added to the culture media were shown to inhibit invasion [34,45]. In experiments in this author's laboratory [46], we used human recombinant TIMP (rTIMP), which was unglycosylated and had a molecular weight of 20,711. The rTIMP showed a similar ability to inhibit the invasion of murine B16 melanoma cells through the amniotic membrane, as did natural TIMP. The injection of rTIMP into C57BL mice (i.p. every 12 hours for 6 days) significantly decreased the number of B16 melanoma tumors formed in the mouse lung after tail-vein injection of the tumor cells. TIMP did not affect the tight binding of the murine melanoma cells to the amniotic membrane, as did the fibronectin (integrin) receptor-binding peptide RDGS and the laminin receptor-binding peptide YIGSR, but instead inhibited invasion of tightly bound cells across the membrane. Furthermore, TIMP had no effect on the size of the tumors formed. In a similar type of experiment with murine B16 melanoma cells, Reich et al. [47] showed that a synthetic collagenase inhibitor inhibits the number of colonies formed in mouse lung from tail-vein injected melanoma cells. These results showing inhibition of lung colonization by both a natural and a synthetic collagenase inhibitor directly support a role for collagenases in the metastasis of tumor cells.

Denhardt and coworkers [48] found that if they downmodulated TIMP synthesis to 50% of its normal level in mouse Swiss 3T3 fibroblasts by expressing an antisense TIMP mRNA, the cells assumed a new phenotype that exhibited an ability to form tumors and metastasize in nude mice. As the normal fibroblasts gave a malignant phenotype on the suppression of TIMP synthesis, TIMP may be a tumor suppressor protein and the TIMP gene may fit the definition of an anti-oncogene. Its expression in the Swiss 3T3 mouse line is apparently required to maintain the normal phenotype. Further experiments in other systems will be required to confirm this intriguing finding.

Recently a second TIMP, designated TIMP-2, has been isolated [49]. The isolation of TIMP-2, homologous to TIMP, indicates that a family of TIMP-related proteins exist. TIMP-2 secreted from human melanoma cells is a 21-kD protein that binds in a 1:1 stoichiometry with the 72-kD type IV pro-collagenase that is also secreted by the same cells. TIMP-2 preferentially interacts with the 72-kD collagenase. The 92-kD type IV collagenase only interacts with TIMP, though TIMP can inhibit both the 92-kD and 72-kD enzymes [50]. A 20-kD type IV collagenase inhibitor, which is not recognized by TIMP antibodies, has recently been purified from bovine aortic endothelial cells [51].

Neutrophil elastase, trypsin, and chymotrypsin were shown to destroy the inhibitory activity of TIMP by degrading the inhibitor into small fragments [52]. Perhaps TIMP is broken down in certain environments by cellular secretions of TIMP-degrading proteases [53].

6.4. Tissue and urokinase type plasminogen activators are also associated with the transformed and metastatic phenotype, and may act by activating the proenzyme forms of metalloproteinases

Evidence for the involvement of the serine-type protease plasminogen activators in cancer cell metastasis is quite extensive [3,54,55]. Plasminogen activator (PA) can act directly to degrade basement membrane proteoglycans and glycoproteins or indirectly by generating active plasmin from its zymogen plasminogen. Plasminogen is found in significant concentrations in extracellular compartments. Perhaps the pertinent observation is that plasmin can activate type IV procollagenases, which can then initiate the degradation of the collagens of the extracellular matrix. Thus, there may exist a proteolytic cascade in which tumor-cell secreted plasminogen activator activates plasmin, which in turn activates extracellular prometalloproteinases [56,57]. Two genetically and immunologically distinct forms of plasminogen activator are known, urokinase and tissue plasminogen activator. In most cases, the plasminogen activator increased with transformation is found to be the urokinase type rather than the tissue plasminogen activator type [55]. Paranjpe et al. [56] early suggested the activation of human breast carcinoma procollagenase by plasminogen activator. He et al. [57] demonstrated that in cocultures of keratinocytes and skin fibroblasts, both type I procollagenase and prostromelysin have a plasmin-dependent activation. Plasmin generated an active type I collagenase by cleaving approximately 80 amino acids from the NH_2-terminal end of the procollagenase. Catalytic amounts of stromelysin, in turn, convert plasmin-activated collagenase into a fully active enzyme by removing an additional 15 amino acid residues from its COOH-terminal end. The fully activated enzyme has a five- to eightfold higher activity than the partially activated enzyme [57]. Stromelysin alone could not activate procollagenase [57].

Ossowski and Reich have reported that an antibody to human urokinase injected into a chick embryo will significantly inhibit the metastasis to the chick embryo lung of human HEp3 epidermal carcinoma cells placed on the chick embryo chorioallantoic membrane [58]. Recent work in this laboratory [59] and by Axelrod et al. [60] show that expression of human prourokinase in transformed murine cells transfected with the human preprourokinase gene will significantly increase the ability of these cells to metastasize. The increased urokinase expression also apparently leads to a higher collagenase activity in culture [60], supporting the hypothesis that the relationship between the higher urokinase activity and metastatic ability is due to a role of urokinase in the activation of procollagenases.

7. Possible cooperation between malignant cells and normal cells in the induction of metalloproteinase activities

An alternate or coinciding hypothesis to the contention that malignant cells synthesize and secrete their own collagenolytic matrix degrading activity is that they induce host cells to produce degradative enzymes. Biswas and Nugent [61] have shown that tumor cells can make a factor, called collagenase stimulatory factor (CSF), that causes fibroblasts to secrete collagenases. Bauer et al. [62] noted a high collagenase activity associated with fibroblasts isolated from human basal cell carcinomas. It was suggested that the tumors may have stimulated adjacent fibroblasts to produce collagenase, which is of importance to the invasion of the tumor. Dabbous et al. [63] reported an increase in mast cells within zones of tumor invasion. It was suggested that mast cells may act as helper cells to metastasis and may induce collagenase synthesis in host fibroblasts and in tumor cells.

8. Induction of metalloproteinase activities by exogenous factors

Many tumor cells metastasize to only certain organs or tissues, and there must exist certain environmental signals that induce a particular tumor to invade and form metastases in a particular target tissue. These signals or factors that modulate the metastatic phenotype in vivo have not been clearly identified. In addition to collagenase stimulatory factor, other factors that may control metalloproteinase and metalloproteinase inhibitor gene expressions have been studied in vitro, and it is assumed these same factors or factors like them may act in vivo within the microenvironment of the metastasizing tumor cell.

Retinoids have been shown to increase TIMP synthesis two- to threefold in cultured human fibroblasts with a simultaneous two- to threefold decrease in type I collagenase synthesis [64]. Dexamethasone causes a dose-dependent decrease in collagenase without altering the biosynthesis of TIMP in the human fibroblasts [64].

Tumor necrosis factor-*alpha*, which is secreted by macrophages in response to inflammation, infection, and cancer, was shown to stimulate tupe I collagenase transcription in human AF2 fibroblasts [65]. Tumor growth factor-*beta* was shown to decrease type I collagenase activity, but to increase TIMP and type IV collagenase synthesis in quiescent human fibroblasts [66]. Transcription from the stromelysin promoter is induced by IL-1 and is repressed by dexamethasone [67,68].

In cultured SV-40 transformed fibroblasts, the expression of metalloproteinase genes was shown to be upregulated by phorbol esters, cAMP, growth factors, IL-1, calcium ionophores, agents remodeling the actin cytoskeleton, and agents causing transformation. The metalloproteinase genes were downregulated by glucocorticoids and retinoids. TIMP was regulated independently. Phorbol ester and IL-1 upregulated TIMP, as it did the metalloproteinases. However, retinoids, transformation agents, and cytoskeletal regulators downregulated TIMP gene expression [69].

Upregulation of the type I collagenase gene by the oncogene products of v-*src*, c-Ha-*ras*, activated c-Ha-*ras*, and v-*mos*, as well as phorbol esters, was shown to require c-*fos* gene expression in murine NIH 3T3 cells [70]. The importance of c-Fos in stimulation of stromelysin by PDGF but not EGF was reported by Kerr et al. [71].

Edwards et al. [72] showed that the exposure of quiescent MRC-5 human fibroblasts to epidermal growth factor, basic fibroblast growth factor, or embryonal-carcinoma-derived growth factor resulted in an increase in the mRNA for type I collagenase, stromelysin, and TIMP. The exposure of the cells to these growth factors in the presence of tumor growth factor-*beta* resulted in the inhibition of the collagenase mRNA induction, but, in contrast, caused the synergistic increase in TIMP mRNA. The result shows that TGFβ has a selective effect on metalloproteinase and TIMP gene expressions in MRC-5 fibroblasts.

9. Surface metalloproteinase activity

Kramer et al. [73] reported that murine B16 melanoma cells required tumor cell contact with extracellular matrix in order to solubilize the matrix components in an in vitro assay. The location in the plasma membrane of metalloproteinase activities able to degrade collagens and fibronectin, and correlated with metastatic potential, has been reported [74–78]. It is suggested that these cell surface metalloproteinases have a role in tumor cell migrations. However, these enzymes must be purified, and more specific data on the characterization of their activities must be obtained before their possible functions are known.

10. Conclusions

There exist a significant number of papers showing correlations between metastatic ability and increases in metalloproteinase activity, especially type IV collagenolytic activity. In addition, a positive correlation exists between plasminogen activator activity and metastatic potential. Metastatic tumor cells may thus secrete high amounts of both procollagenase and prourokinase. The activated urokinase initiates an enzymatic cascade, resulting in the initial activation by urokinase of plasminogen and the subsequent activation of prometalloproteinases by plasmin. The activated metalloproteinases degrade extracellular matrix proteins during tumor cell invasion. In addition, urokinase and plasmin may have important activities of their own in the degradation of the extracellular matrix [79]. The action of recombinant TIMP in inhibiting murine experimental metastasis supports the importance of metalloproteinases in metastasis and further indicates a role for metalloproteinase inhibitors in modulating metastasis [46]. A future capacity to either control the activation of the metalloproteinases in the environment of tumor cells or to increase the concentration of metalloproteinase inhibitors in situ may result in an ability to control the metastatic process.

References

1. Liotta, L.A. (1988) Oncogene induction of metastases. In: Metastasis (Ciba Found. Symp. 141), Chichester, John Wiley and Sons, pp. 94–108.
2. Liotta L.A. Rao C.N., Wewer U.M. (1986) Biochemical interactions of tumor cells with basement membrane. Annu. Rev. Biochem. 55:1037–1057.
3. Goldfarb, R.H., and Liotta, L.A. (1986) Proteolytic enzymes in cancer invasion and metastasis. Semin. Thromb. Hemost. 12:294–307.
4. Collier, I.E., Wilhelm, S.M., Eisen, A.Z., Marmer, B.L., Grant, G.A., Seltzer, J.L., Kronberger, A., He, C.S., Bauer, E.A., Goldberg, G.I. (1988) H-*ras* oncogene-transformed human bronchial epithelial cells (TBE-1) secrete a single metalloproteinase capable of degrading basement membrane collagen. J. Biol. Chem. 263:6579–6587.
5. Wilhelm, S.M., Collier, I.E., Marmer, B.L., Eisen, A.Z., Grant, G.A., Goldberg, G.I. (1989) SV-40 transformed human lung fibroblasts secrete a 92 kDalton type IV collagenase which is identical to that secreted by normal human macrophages. J. Biol. Chem. 264:17213–17221.
6. Goldberg, G.I., Wilhelm, S.M., Kronberger, A., Bauer, E.A., Grant, G.A., Eisen, A.Z. (1986) Human fibroblast collagenase. J. Biol. Chem. 261:6600–6605.
7. Saus, J., Quinones, S., Otani, Y., Nagase, H., Harris, E.D. Jr., Kurkinen, M. (1988) The complete primary structure of human matrix metalloproteinase-3. J. Biol. Chem. 263: 6742–6745.
8. Wilhelm, S.C., Collier, I.E., Kronberger, A., Eisen, A.Z., Marmer, B.L., Grant, G.A., Bauer, E.A., Goldberg, G.I. (1987) Human skin fibroblast stromelysin: Structure, glycosylation, substrate specificity, and differential expression in normal and tumorigenic cells. Proc. Natl. Acad. Sci. USA 84:6725–6729.
9. Sirum, K.L., Brinckerhoff, C.E. (1989) Cloning of the genes for human stromelysin and stromelysin 2: Differential expression in rheumatoid synovial fibroblasts. Biochemistry 28:8691–8698.
10. Nakajima, M., Irimura, T., Di Ferrante, N., Nicolson, G.L. (1984) Characterization of heparan sulfate degradation fragments produced by B16 melanoma endoglucuronidase. J. Biol. Chem. 259:2283–2290.
11. Gunja-Smith, Z., Nagase, H., Woessner, J.F., Jr. (1989) Purification of the neutral proteoglycan-degrading metalloproteinase from human articular cartilage tissue and its identification as stromelysin matrix metalloproteinase-3. Biochem. J. 258:115–119.
12. Quantin, B., Murphy, G., Breathnach, R. (1989) Pump-1 cDNA codes for a protein with characteristics similar to those of classical collagenase family members. Biochem. 28: 5327–5334.
13. Chin, J.R., Murphy, G., Werb, Z. (1985) Stromelysin, a connective tissue-degrading metalloendopeptidase secreted by stimulated rabbit synovial fibroblasts in parallel with collagenase. J. Biol. Chem. 260:12367–12376.
14. Yurchenco, P.D., Ruben, G.C. (1987) Basement membrane structure in situ: Evidence for lateral associations in the type IV collagen network. J. Cell Biol. 105:2559–2568.
15. Martin, G.R., Timpl, R., (1987) Laminin and other basement membrane components. Annu. Rev. Cell Biol. 3:57–85.
16. Wewer, U.M., Taraboletti, G., Sobel, M.E., Albrechtsen, R., Liotta, L.A. (1987) Role of laminin receptor in tumor cell migration. Cancer Res. 47:5691–5698.
17. Iwamoto, Y., Robey, F.A., Graf, J., Sasaki, M., Kleinman, H.K., Yamada, Y., Martin, G.R. (1987) YIGSR, a synthetic laminin pentapeptide inhibits experimental metastasis formation. Science 238:1132–1134.
18. Mosher, D.F., ed. (1989) Fibronectin, Biology of Extracellular Matrix: A Series, Academic Press, San Diego.
19. Hynes R.O. (1987) Integrins: A family of cell surface receptors. Cell 48:549–554.
20. Humphries, M.J., Olden, K., Yamada, K.M., (1986) A snythetic peptide from fibronectin

inhibits experimental metastasis of murine melanoma cells. Science 233:467–470.
21. Liotta, L.A., Tryggvason, K., Garbisa, S., Hart, I., Foltz, C.M., Shafie, S. (1980) Metastatic potential correlates with enzymatic degradation of basement membrane collagen. Nature 284:67–68.
22. Garbisa, S., Pozzatti, R., Muschel, R.J., Saffiotti, U., Ballin, M., Goldfarb, R.H., Khoury, G., Liotta, L.A. (1987) Secretion of type IV collagenolytic protease and metastatic phenotype: Induction by transfection with c-Ha-*ras* but not c-Ha-*ras* plus AD2-Ela. Cancer Res. 47:1523–1528.
23. Ballin, M., Gomez, D.E., Sinha, C.C., Thorgeirsson, U.P. (1988) *Ras* oncogene mediated induction of a 92 kDa metalloproteinase; strong correlation with the malignant phenotype. Biochem. Biophys. Res. Commun. 154:832–838.
24. Eisenbach, L., Segal, S., Feldman, M., (1985) Proteolytic enzymes in tumor metastasis. II. Collagenase type IV activity in subcellular fractions of cloned tumor populations. J. Natl. Cancer Inst. 74:87–93.
25. Garbisa, S., de Giovanni, C., Biagini, G., Vasi, V., Grigioni, W.F., Errico, A.D., Mancini, A.M., Del, R.E., B., Lollini, P.L., Nanni, P., Nicoletti, G., Prodi, G. (1988) Different metastatic aggressiveness by murine TS/A clones: Ultrastructure, extracellular glycoproteins and type IV collagenolytic activity. Invasion Metastasis 8:177–192.
26. Matrisian, L.M., Bowden, G.T., Krieg, P., Furstenberger, G., Briand, J.P., Leroy, P., Breathnach, R. (1986) The mRNA coding for the secreted protease transin is expressed more abundantly in malignant than in benign tumors. Proc. Natl. Acad. Sci. USA 83:9413–9417.
27. Ostrowski, L.E., Finch, J., Krieg, P., Matrisian, L., Patskan, G., O'Connell, J.F., Phillips, J., Slaga, T.H., Breathnach, R., Bowden, G.T. (1988) Expression pattern of a gene for a secreted metalloproteinase during late stages of tumor progression. Mol. Cacrinogenesis 1:13–19.
28. Khokha, R., Denhardt, D.T. (1989) Matrix metalloproteinases and tissue inhibitor of metalloproteinases: A review of their role in tumorigenesis and tissue invasion. Invasion Metastasis 9:391–405.
29. Turpeenniemi-Hujanen, T., Thorgeirsson, U.P., Rao, C.N., Liotta L.A. (1986) Laminin increases the release of type IV collagenase from malignant cells. J. Biol. Chem. 261:1883–1880.
30. Werb, Z., Tremble, P.M., Behredtsen, O., Crewley, E., Damsky, C.H. (1989) Signal transduction through the fibronectin receptor induces collagenase and stromelysin gene expression. J. Cell Biology 109:877–889.
31. Terranova, V.P., Maslow, D., Markus, G. (1989) Directed migration of murine and human tumor cells to collagenases and other proteases. Cancer Res. 49:4835–4841.
32. Welgus, H.G., Stricklin, G.P. (1983) Human skin fibroblast collagenase inhibitor; comparative studies in human connective tissues, serum and amniotic fluid. J. Biol. Chem. 258:12259–12264.
33. Liotta, L.A., Thorgeirsson, U.P., Garbisa, S. (1982) Role of collagenases in tumor cell invasion. Cancer Metastasis Rev. 1:277–288.
34. Torgeirsson, U.P., Liotta, L.A., Kalebic, T., Margulies, I.M. Thomas, K., Rios-Candelore, M., Russo, R.G. (1982) Effect of natural protease inhibitors and a chemoattractant on tumor cell invasion in vitro. J. Natl. Cancer Inst. 69:1049–1054.
35. Heath, J.K., Gowen, M., Meikle, M.C., Reynolds, J.J. (1982) Human gingival tissues in culture synthesize three metalloproteinases and a metalloproteinase inhibitor. J. Peridontal Res. 17:183–190.
36. Sellers, A., Murphy, G., Meikle, M.C., Reynolds, J.J. (1979) Rabbit bone collagenase inhibitor blocks the activity of other neutral metalloproteinases. Biochem. Biophys. Res. Commun. 87:581–587.
37. Stricklin, G.P., Welgus, H.G. (1983) Human skin fibroblast collagenase inhibitor. J. Biol. Chem. 258:12252–12258.
38. Enghild, J.J., Salvesen, G., Brew, K., Nagase, H., (1989) Interaction of human rheumatoid

synovial collagenase (matrix metalloproteinase 1) and stromelysin (matrix metalloproteinase 3) with human *alpha* 2-macroglobulin and chicken ovastatin. Binding kinetics and identification of matrix metalloproteinase cleavage sites. J. Biol. Chem. 264:8779–8785.
39. Cooper, T.W., Eisen, A.Z., Stricklin, G.P., Welgus, H.G. (1985) Platelet-derived collagenase inhibitor: Characterization and subcellular location. Proc. Natl. Acad. Sci. USA 82:2779–2783.
40. Wellgus, H.G., Stricklin, G.P. (1983) Human skin fibroblast collagenase inhibitor. J. Biol. Chem. 258:12259–12264.
41. Carmichael, D.F., Sommer, A., Thompson, R.C., Anderson, D.C., Smith, C.G., Welgus, H.G., Stricklin, G.P. (1986) Primary structure and cDNA cloning of human fibroblast collagenase inhibitor. Proc. Natl. Acad. Sci. USA 83:2407–2411.
42. Docherty, A.J.P., Lyons, A., Smith, B.Y., Wright, E.M., Stephens, P.E., Harris, T.J.R., Murphy, G., Reynolds, J.J. (1985) Sequence of human tissue inhibitor of metalloproteinases and its identity to erythroid-potentiating activity. Nature 318:66–69.
43. Gasson, J.C., Golde, D.W., Kaufman, S.E., Westbrook, C.A., Hewick, R.M., Kaufman, R.J., Wong, G.G., Temple, P.A., Leary, A.C., Brown, E.L., Orr, E.C., Clark, S.C. (1985) Molecular characterization and expression of the gene encoding human erythroid-potentiating activity. Nature 315:768–771.
44. Spurr, N.K., Goodfellow, P.N., Docherty, A.J. (1987) Chromosomal assignment of the gene encoding the human tissue inhibitor of metalloproteinases to Xp11.1-p11.4. Ann Hum. Genet. 51:189–194.
45. Mignatti, P., Robbins, E., Rifkin, D.B. (1986) Tumor invasion through the human amniotic membrane: Requirement for a proteinase cascade. Cell 47:487–498.
46. Schultz, R.M., Silberman, S., Persky, B., Bajkowski, A.S., Carmichael, D.F. (1988) Inhibition by human recombinant tissue inhibitor of metalloproteinases of human amnion invasion and lung colonization by murine B16-F10 melanoma cells. Cancer Res. 48: 5539–5545.
47. Reich, R., Thompson, E.W., Iwanoto, Y., Martin, G.R., Deason, J.R., Fuller, G.C., Miskin, R. (1988) Effects of inhibitors of plasminogen activator, serine proteinases, and collagenase IV on the invasion of basement membranes by metastatic cells. Cancer Res. 48:3307–3312.
48. Kjokja, R., Waterhouse, P., Yagel, S., Lala, P.K., Overall, C.M., Norton, G., Denhardt, D.T. (1988) Antisense RNA induced reduction in murine TIMP levels and confers oncogenicity on Swiss 3T3 cells. Science 243:947–950.
49. Stetler-Stevenson, W.G., Krutzsch, H.C., Liotta, L.A. (1989) Tissue inhibitor of metalloproteinase (TIMP-2). J. Biol. Chem. 264:17374–17378.
50. Goldberg, G.I., Marmer, B.L., Grant, G.A., Eisen, A.Z., Wilhelm, S., He., C.(1989) Human 72 kDalton type IV collagenase forms a complex with tissue inhibitor of metalloproteinases designated TIMP-2. Proc. Natl. Acad. Sci. USA 86:8207–8211.
51. de Clerck, Y.A., Yean, T.D., Ratzkin, B.J., Lu., H.S., Langley, K.E. (1989) Purification and characterization of two related but distinct metalloproteinase inhibitors secreted by bovine aortic endothelial cells. J. Biol. Chem. 264:17445–17453.
52. Okada, Y., Watanabe, S., Nakanishi, I., Kishi, J., Ayakawa, T., Watorek, W. (1988) Inactivation of TIMP by neutrophil elastase and other serine proteinases. FEBS Lett. 229:157–160.
53. Ponton, A., Waghorne, C., Coulombe, B., Kerbel, R.S., Breitman, M., Skup, D. (1988) Expression of TIMP gene during formation of metastases. Clin. Exp. Metastasis 12 (Supplement):18–19.
54. Quigley, J.P. (1979) Proteolytic enzymes of normal and malignant cells. In: Hynes, R.O., ed. Surfaces of Normal and Malignant Cells, John Wiley and Sons, New York.
55. Dano, K, Andreasen, P.A., Grondahl-Hansen, J., Kristensen, P., Nielsen, L.S., Skriver, L. (1985) Plasminogen activators, tissue degradation, and cancer. Adv. Cancer Res. 44: 139–266.
56. Paranjpe, M., Engel, L., Young, N., Liotta, L.A. (1980) Activation of human breast

carcinoma collagenase through plasminogen activator. Life Sci. 26:1223–1231.
57. He, C., Wilhelm, S.M., Pentland, A.P., Marmer, B.L., Grant, G.A., Eisen, A.Z., Goldberg, G.I. (1989) Tissue cooperation in a proteolytic cascade activating human interstitial collagenase. Proc. Natl. Acad. Sci. USA 86:2632–2636.
58. Ossowski, L., Reich, E. (1983) Antibodies to plasminogen activator inhibit human tumor metastasis. Cell 35:611–619.
59. Yu, H., Schultz, R.M. (1990) Murine B16-F1 melanoma cells transfected with the human urokinase gene show an increased ability to metastasize, Cancer Res., in press.
60. Axelrod, J.H., Reich, R., Miskin, R. (1989) Expression of human recombinant plasminogen activators enhances invasion and experimental metastasis of H-*ras* transformed NIH 3T3 cells. Mol. Cell. Biol. 9:2133–2141.
61. Biswas, C., Nugent, M.A. (1987) Membrane association of collagenase stimulatory factor(s) from B16 melanoma cells. J. Cell Biochem. 35:247–258.
62. Bauer, E.A., Uitto, J., Walters, R.C., Eisen, A.Z. (1979) Enhanced collagenase production by fibroblasts derived from human basal cell carcinomas. Cancer Res. 39:4594–4599.
63. Dabbous, M.K., Woolley, D.E., Haney, L., Carter, L.M., Nicolson, G.L. (1986) Host mediated effectors of tumor invasion: Role of mast cells in matrix degradation. Clin. Expl. Metastasis 4:141–152.
64. Clark, S.D., Kobayashi, D.K., Welgus, H.G. (1987) Regulation of the expression of tissue inhibitor of metalloproteinases and collagenase by retinoids and glucocorticoids in human fibroblasts. J. Clin. Invest. 80:1280–1288.
65. Brenner, D.A., O'Hara, M., Angel, P., Chojkier, M., Karin, M. (1989) Prolonged activation of Jun and collagenase genes by tumour necrosis factor *alpha*. Nature 337:661–666.
66. Overall, C.M., Wrana, J.L., Sodek, J. (1989) Independent regulation of collagenase 72 kDA progelatinase, and metalloendoproteinase inhibitor expression in human fibroblasts by TGF *beta*. J. Biol. Chem. 264:1860–1869.
67. Frisch, S.M., Ruley, H.E. (1987) Transcription from the stromelysin promoter is induced by interleukin-1 and repressed by dexamethasone. J. Biol. Chem. 262:16300–16304.
68. Quinones, S., Saus, J., Otani, Y., Harris, E.D. Jr., Kurkinen, M. (1989) Transcriptional regulation of human stromelysin. J. Biol. Chem. 264:8339–8344.
69. Werb, Z., Adler, R.A., Behrendtsen, O., Brenner, C.A., Chin, J.R., Clark, E.J., Frisch, S.M., Rappolee, D.A., Tremble, P.M., Unemori, E.N. (1988) Metalloproteinase gene expression in development, differentiation, transformation and disease. J. Cell Biochem. 12B:274.
70. Schonthal, A., Herrlich, P., Rahmsdorf, H.J., Ponta, H. (1988) Requirement for c-*fos* protooncogene expression in the transcriptional activation of collagenases by other oncogenes and phorbol esters. Cell 54:325–334.
71. Kerr, L.D., Holt, J.T., Matrisian, L.M. (1988) Growth factors regulate transin gene expression by c-*fos*-dependent and c-*fos*-independent pathways. Science 242:1424–1427.
72. Edwards, D.R., Murphy, G., Reynolds, J.J., Whitham, S.E., Docherty, A.J., Angel, P., Heath, J.K. (1987) Transforming growth factor *beta* modulates the expression of collagenase and metalloproteinase inhibitor. EMBO J. 6:1899–1904.
73. Kramer, R.H., Vogel, K.G., Nicolson, G.L. (1982) Solubilization and degradation of subendothelial matrix glycoproteins and proteoglycans by metastatic tumor cells. J. Biol. Chem. 257.2678–2686.
74. Zucker, S., Wieman, J.M., Lysik, R.M., Wilkie, D., Ramamurthy, N.S., Golub, L.M., Lane, B. (1987), Enrichment of collagen and gelatin degrading activities in the plasma membranes of human cancer cells. Cancer Res. 47:1608–1614.
75. Zucker, S., Lysik, R.M., Wieman, J., Wilkie, D.P., Lane, B. (1985) Diversity of human pancreatic cancer cell proteinases: Role of cell membrane metalloproteinases in collagenolysis and cytolysis. Cancer Res. 45:6168–6178.
76. Chen, W.T., Olden, K., Bernard, B.A., Chu, F.F. (1984) Expression of transformation-associated proteases that degrade fibronectin at cell contact sites. J. Cell Biol. 98:1546–1555.
77. Chen, J.M., Chen, W.T. (1987) Fibronectin degrading proteases from the membranes of

transformed cells. Cell 48:193–203.
78. Werb, Z., Clark, E.J. (1989) Phorbol diesters regulate expression of the membrane neutral metalloendopeptidase (EC 3.4.24.11) in rabbit synovial fibroblasts and mammary epithelial cells. J. Biol. Chem. 264:9111–9113.
79. Sullivan, L.M., Quigley, J.P. (1986) An anticatalytic monoclonal antibody to avian plasminogen activator: Its effect on behavior of RSV-transformed chick fibroblasts. Cell 45:905–915.

IV

Antigens

8. Ganglioside antigens in tissue sections of skin, naevi, and melanoma — Implications for treatment of melanoma

Peter Hersey

1. Introduction

Ganliosides were first described by Ernst Klenk in 1936 as a class of glycolipid-containing sialic acids that were found in brain tissue [1]. It is now known that they are components of cells in most tissues and that they are synthesized by glycosyltransferases in the plasma membrane, Golgi apparatus, and microsomes of cells [1,2]. They appear to serve as receptors for products such as cholera and tetanus toxin [2], viruses [3,4], and hormones, such as thyroid-stimulating hormone [2], serotonin [2], interleukin-2 (IL-2) [5], and interferon [2]. They appear to have an important role in cell membranes in either enhancing [6] or inhibiting signal transduction resulting from receptor interactions with a variety of growth factors, such as epidermal growth factor, fibroblast growth factor, and platelet-derived growth factors [6–8]. In some tissues they appear to be associated with activation of Ca^{2+}-dependent protein kinases [9] and Ca^{2+}-flux across cell membranes [10].

Malignant melanoma is known to express a number of gangliosides that are not detected in normal melanocytes. In this sense they can therefore be regarded as tumor-associated neoantigens [11]. When compared to brain, melanoma has much less of the complex ganliosides — GT1, GD1, and GM1 — and higher concentrations of the simpler gangliosides — GM3, GM2, and GD3, and to a lesser extent, GD2 [11–13]. More recently gangliosides with O-acetylated sialic acids [14] and N-glycolyl sialic acids [11] have been identified in melanoma. The former appear specific to melanoma, whereas the latter are also found in red blood cells from other species [15]. Monoclonal antibodies (MAbs) have been produced against a number of gangliosides expressed on human melanoma cells, including those against GD3 [12,16], GD2 [17,18], GM3 [19], and GM2 [20,21]. Interest in the clinical use of these MAbs was stimulated by reports that the injection of MAb against GD3 or GD2 into patients with melanoma induced remissions in tumor growth [22–24]. Intralesional injections of human MAb against GD2 were also reported to induce the regression of subcutaneous metastatic melanoma [25].

These clinical responses following the injection of MAbs to gangliosides were of particular interest, as the treatment of patients with (unconjugated)

L. Nathanson (ed.), MELANOMA RESEARCH: GENETICS, GROWTH FACTORS, METASTASES, AND ANTIGENS.

MAbs against other melanoma-associated antigens did not induce regression of tumor growth [26–28]. These differences in clinical responses were not accounted for by differences in antibody class or in the density of the antigen on the melanoma cell surface [29]. Studies by ourselves [30,31] and others [32] have suggested that one of the reasons for this may be the ability of MAbs against certain gangliosides to potentiate or activate immune responses due to their interaction with gangliosides on activated lymphocytes. These findings, therefore, raised the possibility that their effects on tumor growth may have been indirect and due to stimulation of immune responses of the host against their function.

In addition to their interest as targets for the treatment with MAbs, several studies have suggested that certain of the gangliosides may be immunogenic in their hosts [33]. In particular, antibodies against GD2 were reported in patients with melanoma [34,35], and the generation of such responses was suggested to be associated with a good prognosis [36]. Portoukalian et al. [37] also reported IgG antibody responses to a number of different gangliosides in patients treated with vaccines containing a mixture of gangliosides and suggested this response was associated with a favorable prognosis.

In view of their potential as targets for MAbs or as vaccines, studies were carried out to study the distribution of three of the major gangliosides in melanoma and on lymphocytes in tissue sections of melanoma. The present chapter describes the results of these studies and discusses some of the functional effects that might be expected from the interaction of MAbs with melanoma and lymphocytes in vivo.

2. Distribution of gangliosides GD3, GD2, and GM3 on melanocytes, naevi, and melanoma

Analysis of tissue sections of melanoma with MAbs against GD3, GD2, and GM3 were carried out using immunoperoxidase techniques. Studies were carried out on normal skin, 19 naevi, 29 primaries, and 83 metastases [38]. The results of these studies can be summarized as follows.

The ganglioside GD3 appeared to be expressed on all melanocytic tissues studied, including melanocytes, naevi, and primary and metastatic melanoma. Expression of GD3 was not uniform in the tumors, and in most of the sections GD3-negative tumor cells could be identified. This is shown by the histograms in Figure 1.

GM3 was not identified on melanocytes, even though this ganglioside was reported to be found in extracts of cultured melanocytes [18]. It was present on cells in naevi, but was noticeably absent when naevus cells were located in the epidermis, in compound or junctional naevi. As shown in Figure 1, GM3 was detected on 63% of primary and 75% of metastatic melanomas. The expression of GM3 on cells in individual tumors was lower than that of GD3 and, as noted in naevi, GM3 was absent from tumor cells located in the epidermis.

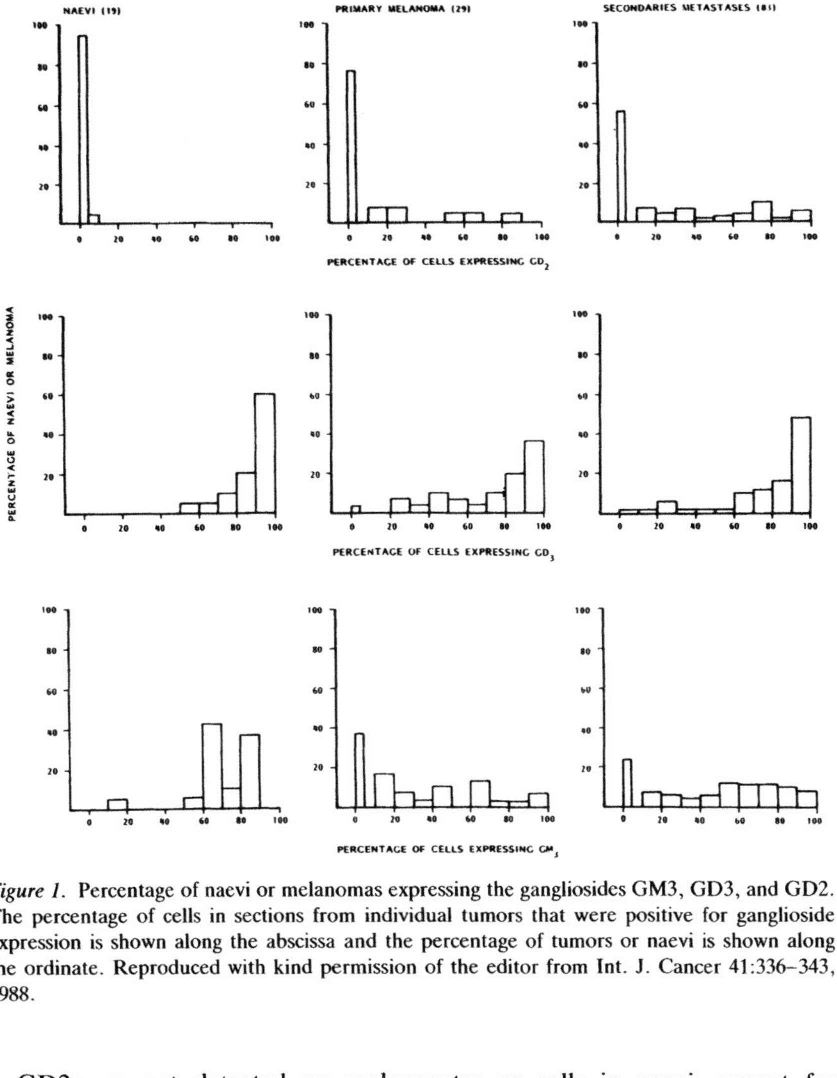

Figure 1. Percentage of naevi or melanomas expressing the gangliosides GM3, GD3, and GD2. The percentage of cells in sections from individual tumors that were positive for ganglioside expression is shown along the abscissa and the percentage of tumors or naevi is shown along the ordinate. Reproduced with kind permission of the editor from Int. J. Cancer 41:336–343, 1988.

GD3 was not detected on melanocytes or cells in naevi, except for occasional areas of so-called neuroidal differentiation of naevus cells deep in the dermis. As shown in Figure 1, GD2 was detected on a low percentage of tumor cells in approximately 25% of primary melanomas and in approximately 45% of metastases.

2.1. Interrelationship between GM3, GD3, and GD2 expression on melanoma

In view of the biosynthetic pathway described by Fishman and Brady [2], a reciprocal relationship might be expected between the expression of GM3 and GD3, or GD3 and GD2. Regression analysis, as shown in Figure 2, suggested instead that GM3 and GD3, and GD3 and GD2, tended to be

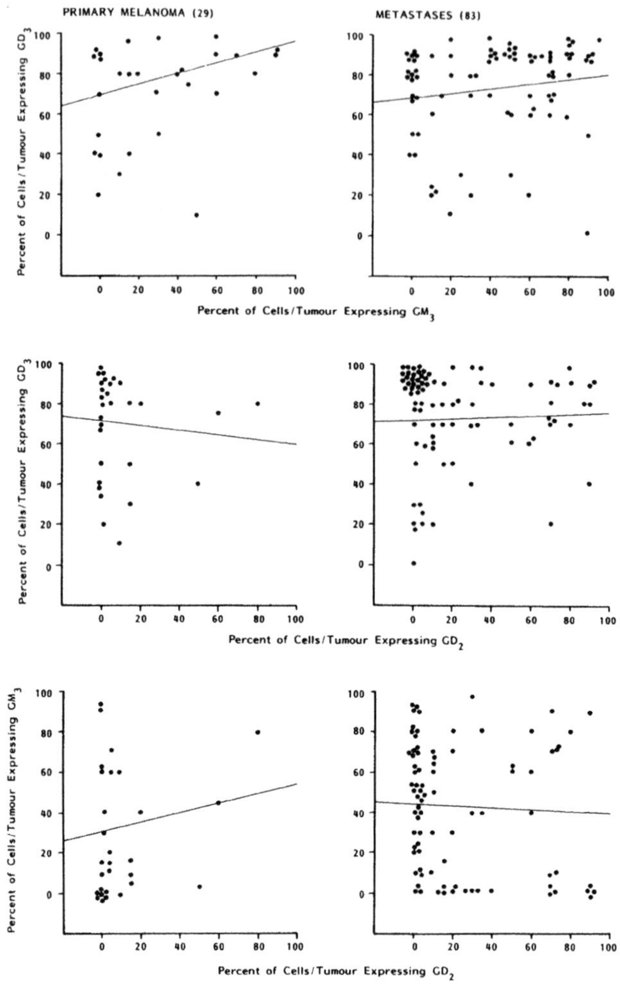

Figure 2. Relation between expression of GD3, GM3, and GD2 on primary and metastatic melanoma. Regression equation for GD3 vs. GM3 expression on primary melanomas was GD3 = 63.4 + 0.339 GM3 (t = 2.39) and on metastatic melanomas was GD3 = 66.4 + 0.138 GM3 (t = 1.53 ns). Reproduced with kind permission of the editor from Int. J. Cancer 41: 336–343, 1988.

coexpressed on melanoma cells. There was no correlation between GM3 or GD3 expression with that of GD2 expression. However, it is possible that analysis in this way may give a false impression if there were mixed populations of tumors, e.g., the data relating GM3 to GD2 expression could be interpreted to suggest two populations were present — one in which GM3 and GD2 were negatively related and a second in which both GM3 and GD2 are coexpressed.

Studies on primary melanoma and metastases from individual patients shown in Table 1 provided some evidence for a reciprocal relationship between GD3 and GD2, in that when metastatic lesions had an increase in the percentage of cells expressing GD2, there was a decrease in the percentage of cells expressing GD3 relative to that on primaries. Conversely, when the primary tumor had cells expressing GD2 but the metastasis did not, there was an increase in the percentage of cells expressing GD3 in the metastasis.

2.2. *GD2 and malignant potential*

Several reports suggest that the expression of GD2 on primary melanoma was associated with metastatic potential [39], and in particular that its expression was related to the vertical growth phase, rather than the radial growth phase, of melanoma [11,18]. This could not be confirmed in our series in that 4 of 13 in the vertical and 2 of 11 primary melanomas in the radial growth phase expressed GD2 [38]. Moreover, although there was a higher incidence of GD2 expression on metastases, over half of the latter had no detectable GD2. This would imply that GD2 is not essential to the metastatic process and the presence or absence of GD2 on primary melanoma cannot be taken as a guide to its metastatic potential. To emphasize this point we also found no correlation with thickness of the primary melanoma

Table 1. Expression of gangliosides on primary and metastatic melanoma from individual patients

Patient	MAb	Primary % positive	Metastases % positive
MA	GM3	90	2
	GD3	95	25
	GD2	2	30
MP	GM3	60	5
	GD3	70	25
	GD2	0	20
NC	GM3	60	70
	GD3	60	10
	GD2	10	50
JN	GM3	2	70
	GD3	50	60
	GD2	0	0
DS	GM3	30	30
	GD3	50	95
	GD2	50	0
KR	GM3	5	50
	GD3	90	90
	GD2	0	0

Values indicated are percentage of cells positive in each section.
Reproduced with kind permission of the editor from Int. J. Cancer 41:336–343, 1988.

(if anything, there was an inverse correlation), which is accepted to be the most reliable indicator of prognosis [38].

It was also analyzed whether particular patterns of ganglioside expression may determine the site of metastases. There was no evidence from this analysis that expression of GD3, GM3, or GD2 had any association with metastases in lymph nodes (LNs) or subcutaneous sites.

2.3. *Tissue-dependent changes in ganglioside expression*

It was noted during these studies that the distribution of gangliosides appeared to be influenced by adjacent tissues, e.g., GD3 was not expressed on epithelial cells in normal skin but was expressed on epithelial cells in the stratum spinosum above naevi and primary melanoma. Similarly, GM3 was not expressed on naevus cells or melanoma cells when these were located in the epidermis, even though it was expressed on cells in the same naevi or melanoma in regions located in the dermis. GD2 was expressed around epithelial cells in the basal layer and to a lesser extent in the stratum spinosum, especially near hair follicles in normal skin. This pattern of staining was much more intense above naevi, but was absent in epithelium adjacent to or above primary melanoma [38].

These tissue-dependent changes may suggest that chemical factors released from naevus or melanoma cells act to regulate the glycosyl transferase enzymes involved in the synthesis of GD3 and GD2, e.g., Rosenberg et al. [40] reported that increased GD3 synthesis in melanoma reflected an increase in GD3 synthetase enzyme levels and not a deficiency of enzymes further on in the synthetic chain [2]. The absence of GM3 expression in cells from naevi and melanoma located in the epidermis is more difficult to explain and suggests a negative regulatory influence by the keratinocytes or consumption of GM3 for GD3 synthesis.

2.4. *Therapeutic implications*

The results from these studies on tissue sections suggested that MAbs directed against GD3 would interact with the highest proportion of melanoma cells in the highest proportion of melanomas in patients. The specificity of these antibodies also appeared high in that they reacted with very few normal tissues. In skin reactivity was mainly against melanocytes, fibroblasts, and reticular tissue around blood vessels, and some lymphocytes. In LNs there was reactivity with reticular cells lining the framework and around blood vessels [44]. MAbs against GM3 also had very little reactivity with nonmelanoma tissues and did not react with any of the normal tissues in skin or LNs. MAbs to GD2 reacted with peripheral nerves, as well as epithelial cells, in skin, as described above. They also showed marked reactivity with lymphocytes in LNs, as described below. Although MAbs to GD3, and to a lesser extent GM3, reacted with a high percentage of tumors, the percentage of cells in each tumor that reacted with the MAbs was variable. At least half the tumors contained some GD3-negative cells and 90% of tumors contained GM3-negative cells. This would imply that residual foci of cells would be left after treatment with the MAbs.

Another pertinent question is whether a combination of MAbs to GD3 and GM3 would be more effective than either above. The regression analysis in Figure 2 suggested this may not be so, in that tumors tended to have coordinate expression of both gangliosides. With few exceptions, cells positive for GM3 were also positive for GD3. Nevertheless, the use of both MAbs may increase their damaging effect on an individual cell basis.

The same considerations apply to use of MAbs against GD2 in that GD2-negative tumor cells were apparent in practically all melanomas. Combination of antibodies against GD3 and GD2 may, however, increase reactivity with cells in individual tumors in that reciprocal expression of GD2 and GD3 was apparent in areas of individual tumors.

In view of these findings on tissue sections, it is somewhat surprising that treatment with MAbs to GD3 and GD2 have been as effective as reported. These studies are summarized in Table 2. This is even more so when these results are compared to the negative results from treatment with MAbs against other antigens on melanoma cells that have an equal or wider distribution on melanoma than that of the gangliosides [27,28].

We have suggested that one of the explanations for this may be activation of T-cell responses of the host against the tumor by the MAbs, i.e., the effects of the MAbs on tumors is indirect via the immune response of the host. We have previously reported that MAbs to GD3 and GD2 potentiated lymphocyte responses to a number of stimuli, including melanoma antigens [30,31]. These studies also showed that blood lymphocytes expressed GD3 when they were activated [30,44]. To sustain the hypothesis that the MAbs were able to interact with lymphocytes in vivo, it was necessary to demonstrate that lymphocytes around melanomas expressed gangliosides on their surface. The studies below summarize the evidence for this.

3. Ganglioside expression on lymphocytes and melanoma in skin and lymph nodes

This question was analyzed by immunoperoxidase methods on sections from 16 primary melanomas, 10 subcutaneous melanomas, and 22 lymph node (LN) metastases [44]. As shown in Table 3, lymphocytes around the margins of metastases in LNs and in lymphoid follicles next to the metastases frequently expressed GD2. Expression of GD2 was not seen in normal LNs and was infrequent on lymphocytes in the cortex of LNs away from the site of metastases. Subset analysis by dual staining techniques and by the examination of serial sections is summarized in Table 4. This revealed that

Table 2. Unconjugated monoclonal antibody treatment of melanoma

Author	M.Ab	M.A.A.	Total dose	Patients	Results	Site
Houghton et al. [22]	R24 (IgG3)	GD3	8–240 mg/m^2	12	3 PR 2 MR	s.c. LN Lung
Goodman et al. [27]	96.5 (IgG2a) 48.7 (Ig1)	p 97 P.G.	424 mg (212 mg each MAb)	5	PD	
Schroff et al. [28]	9.2.27 (IgG2a)	P.G.	10–200 mg	24	PD	
Goodman et al. [41]	MG21 (IgG3)	GD3	5–100 mg/m^2 daily × 7	8	PD	
Cheung et al. [24]	3F8 (IgG3)	GD2	5–100 mg/m^2	17	7	
Vadhan-Raj et al. [23]	R24 (IgG3)	GD3	1, 10, 30, 50 mg/m/day × 8 doses	21	4 PR 1 MR	
Bajorin et al. [42]	R24 (IgG3)	GD3	1, 3, 8, 12 mg/m^2 daily × 5 + **IL-2**	20	1 PR 2 MR	
Lichtin et al. [43]	ME36.1 (Ig2a)	GD2+GD3	5, 10, 20, 50 mg/m^2 daily × 5	13	1 CR	
Irie et al. [25]	L72 (HuIgM)	GD2	Intralesional 100μg/mm diameter	8	4 PR 2 SD 2 PD	

P.G. = high mol. wt. proteoglycan; p 97 = iron binding protein of 97 kD; MR = mixed response; PR = partial response; PD = progressive disease.

Table 3. Percentage expression of GD2 and GD3 and other markers on lymphocytes in lymph nodes containing metastatic melanoma

	Expression in different anatomical locations (mean ± ISD)				
Lymphocyte marker	Margins of tumor (19)[a]	Tumor infiltrate (18)	Adjacent cortex (17)	Lymphoid follicles (15)	Overall (22)
Lymphocytes $\times 10^{-3}$/mm^2	9.5 ± 2.8	0.27 ± 0.4	11.17 ± 1.3	7.4 ± 0.8	7.2 ± 0.9
GD2 (14.18)	53 ± 27 [0.021][b]	32 ± 37 [0.05]	10 ± 8 [0.53]	55 ± 38 [0.001]	9 ± 5
GD3 (R24)	31 ± 28	11 ± 26	12 ± 14	5 ± 10	13 ± 12
CD4 (Leu3a)	47 ± 15	53 ± 11	47 ± 14	16 ± 8	48 ± 13
CD8 (OKT8)	27 ± 12	31 ± 12	20 ± 12	3 ± 3%	30 ± 16
CD19 (HD37)	26 ± 17	16 ± 14	33 ± 20	79 ± 5	21 ± 13

[a] Figures in parentheses indicate the number of cases with lymphoid infiltrate at these sites.
[b] p values from t tests for comparison of GD2 versus GD3 expression are shown in the brackets.
Reproduced with kind permission of the editor from Pathology 21:51–58, 1989.

Table 4. Percentage expression of gangliosides GD3 and GD on subpopulations of lymphocytes in lymph nodes

Lymphocyte subpopulations	Tumor Margins[a]	Within tumor	Adjacent cortex	Lymphoid follicles
$CD4^+$ $GD2^+$	44 ± 34 (17)[b]	15 ± 29 (15)	10 ± 10 (10)	54 ± 35 (10)
$CD4^+$ $GD3^+$	24 ± 26 (10)	7 ± 14 (14)	14 ± 13 (13)	1 ± 2 (10)
$CD8^+$ $GD2^+$	48 ± 39 (17)	9 ± 15 (15)	13 ± 13 (10)	–
$CD8^+$ $GD3^+$	32 ± 34 (10)	6 ± 12 (14)	14 ± 11 (12)	–
$CD19^+$ $GD2^+$	13 ± 17 (16)	16 ± 32 (12)	16 ± 27 (10)	67 ± 34 (10)
$CD19^+$ $GD3^+$	3 ± 4 (9)	9 ± 29 (12)	13 ± 29 (11)	1 ± 2 (10)

[a] GD2 expression on $CD4^+$ T-cells was significantly above that of GD3 on $CD4^+$ T-cells by a t test of the data ($p < 0.05$ by t test).
[b] Figures in brackets indicate the number of cases studied.
Reproduced with kind permission of the editor from Pathology 21:51–58, 1989.

the GD2-positive lymphocytes around the margins of metastases were mainly $CD4^+$, but $CD8^+$ T-cells also expressed GD2. In the germinal centers of lymphoid follicles, GD2 was expressed predominantly on $CD4^+$ T-cells, B-lymphocytes, and dendritic cells.

GD3 expression on lymphocytes was difficult to assess around tumor margins, because most of the metastases were strongly GD3 positive. The estimates shown in Tables 3 and 4 were made from T200 staining of sections and careful examination under high magnification. GD3 was expressed on lymphocytes in lymphoid follicles, but this was not as marked as GD2 expression. Dual staining and study of serial section showed that GD3 was expressed equally on $CD4^+$ and $CD8^+$ T-cells around the tumor margins and lymphoid follicles. GD3 was also expressed on $CD4^+$ T-cells in the cortex. This subset appeared to have a different distribution from the $CD4^+$ $GD2^+$ T-cells that were located in germinal centers and margins of the metastases.

Expression of gangliosides on lymphocytes in and around primary melanoma and metastases in skin differed from that seen in LNs in that GD2 expression was infrequent and was mainly associated with clusters of $CD4^+$ T-cells at these sites. These studies are summarized in Tables 5 and 6. The $CD4^+$ T-cells did not react with MAbs to CD45R (2H4) but were Leu 8^+, which was reputed to identify a suppressor inducer subset in blood lymphocytes [45]. As these $CD4^+$ T-cells did not express GD2, these results did not suggest any clear association of GD2 expression with suppressor functions of lymphocytes. The studies did not exclude, however, that $CD4^+$

Table 5. Expression of gangliosides GD3 and GD2 on lymphocytes around primary and subcutaneous metastatic melanoma

	Number studied	Lymphocyte count × 10^{-3}/mm^2	GD2 (14.18)	GD3 (R24)	CD4 (Leu3a)	CD8 (OKT8)	CD19 (HD37)
Primary melanoma	16	6.4 ± 3.2	< 1% (11)[a]	9 ± 9[c] (11)	54 ± 11[d] (16)	42 ± 11 (16)	3.4 ± 5 (7)
Subcutaneous metastases	10	8.1 ± 2.1	15 ± 6[b] (5)	26 ± 15 (5)	46 ± 1 (6)	50 ± 3 (6)	4 ± 3 (4)

[a] Figures in brackets indicate the number of cases expressing the marker.
[b] The percentage of lymphocytes in primary melanoma expressing GD2 was significantly less than that around subcutaneous metastases by a t test of the data ($p < 0.05$).
[c] GD3 expression significantly greater than GD2 expression on lymphocytes below primary melanoma (0.003) by t test.
[d] CD4 expression significantly reater than CD8 expression ($p < 0.004$) by t test.
Reproduced with kind permission of the editor from Pathology 21:51–58, 1989.

Table 6. Expression of gangliosides GD3 and GD2 on subpopulations of lymphocytes around primary and subcutaneous metastatic melanoma

	$CD4^+$ $GD2^+$	$CD4^+$ $GD3^+$	$CD8^+$ $GD2^+$	$CD8^+$ $GD3^+$	CD19 GD2
Primary melanoma	< 1% (11)[a]	7 ± 7[b] (14)	< 1% (11)	7 ± 6 (14)	< 1% (8)
Subcutaneous metastases	16 ± 7 (5)	22 ± 20 (5)	10 ± 5 (5)	22 ± 15 (5)	28 ± 43 (5)

[a] Figures in brackets indicate the number of cases expressing the marker.
[b] $CD4^+$ $GD3^+$ ve lymphocytes significantly greater than $CD4^+$ $GD2^+$ ve lymphocytes in primary melanoma ($p < 0.001$).
Reproduced with kind permission of the editor from Pathology 21:51–58, 1989.

$GD3^+$ T-cells may have such a role, and further studies are needed to examine this. GM3 was not detected on lymphocytes.

3.1. Therapeutic implications of GD3 and GD2 expression on lymphocytes

It is apparent from these results that lymphocytes expressing the gangliosides GD3 and GD2 are strategically located near melanoma so that augmentation of their function by MAbs may enhance their antitumor effects against melanoma. It is also clear that if the MAbs did augment lymphocyte function, the outcome may depend on the function of the lymphocytes expressing the gangliosides. In LNs, GD2 appeared to be expressed on lymphocyte subsets involved in antibody production (dendritic cells, $CD4^+$ T-cells, and B-lymphocytes) so that stimulation with MAb to GD2 may enhance antibody production. If the $CD4^+$ T-cells were inducers of suppression, however, the opposite may occur. Similar considerations apply to the effect of MAbs to GD3. In vitro the latter appeared to enhance the cytotoxic activity of CTL [31], but whether the latter occurs in vivo is as yet unproven.

It might also be expected that metastases in skin would not respond as well to treatment with MAbs to GD2, compared to those against GD3, as there were very few lymphocytes in skin expressing GD2. The sites of clinical responses to treatment with MAbs to GD3 were mostly in skin, but a response was also reported in lymph nodes and in lung [22,23]. Inflammatory responses in the skin, particularly around metastases, were a prominent feature in patients treated with these MAbs, which would be consistent with stimulation of T-lymphocytes at these sites by the MAbs. The sites of responses of patients treated with MAbs to GD2 were not stated in the published reports [24]. An interesting side effect noted during treatment with the latter was pain in the extremities, which may reflect the expression of GD2 noted on peripheral nerves.

3.2. Mechanism of potentiation of lymphocyte responses by MAbs to GD2 and GD3

The proliferative response of T-cells to antigens is known to be dependent on the production of IL-2 and receptors for IL-2 (IL-2R), and these two factors were postulated to determine the magnitude of T-cell responses to antigens [45,46]. Analysis of the effects of the MAbs on these two events revealed, firstly, that the MAbs did not have significant effects on IL-2 receptor expression measured by MAbs to Tac. However, the MAbs appeared to increase the affinity of binding of radiolabeled IL-2 to the IL-2R and increased internalization of the latter. Secondly, although the MAbs potentiated phytohemagglutinin (PHA)-induced IL-2 production at high concentrations of MAbs and of PHA, this did not appear to explain their potentiation of the proliferative responses of lymphocytes, e.g., although IL-2 production was minimal or absent from the $CD8^+$ subset, the latter showed the highest degree of augmentation. Addition of IL-2 to PHA-stimulated cultures did not produce similar augmentation of mitogenic responses to that produced by the MAb to GD3 or GD2. The augmented and normal mitogenic responses were, however, dependent on IL-2, as shown by their inhibition with MAbs against IL-2 [47]. These results suggested that the effects of the MAbs on IL-2 production could be distinguished from their effects on the proliferative responses of T-cells and that the latter were associated with changes in affinity and internalization of ^{125}I-IL-2. Whether the latter is a direct cause of the increased proliferative response remains unknown. Studies were also carried out on biochemical changes in lymphocytes induced by MAbs to GD3 and GD2 to determine if these would provide further understanding of the mechanism of the augmented responses. Binding of MAbs to lymphocytes did not appear to be associated with changes in intracellular Ca^{2+} levels, but effects on cell division were associated with increased cyclic GMP levels in lymphocytes. Increases in IL-2 production, on the other hand, appeared to be related to activation of protein kinase C [48].

It is clear from these studies that, quite apart from their potential in the treatment of patients with melanoma, MAbs to GD3 and GD2 may be useful probes to understand the role of these gangliosides in the activation of lymphocytes. If our suggestion that the therapeutic effects of the MAbs are mediated through their effects on lymphocytes is true, the understanding of this role may have important practical applications in treatment.

4. Summary

The ganglioside GD3 was distributed widely on melanocytes, naevi, and practically all melanomas. Not all the cells in melanoma appeared to express GD3, so that treatment with MAbs to GD3 could be expected to leave foci of tumor cells resistant to the effects of the MAbs. GM3 had a similar distribution of GD3 on melanoma, but was expressed on a lower percentage of cells in individual tumors. Expression of GM3 appeared to be suppressed on melanoma and naevus cells in the epidermis. Addition of MAbs to GM3 to those against GD3 in the treatment of melanoma may increase the lytic effect against cells coexpressing both gangliosides, but as GM3 did not appear to be expressed on GM3 -ve cells, the percentage of resistant cells may not be decreased. GD2 was expressed on only approximately 25% of primaries and less than 50% of metastases. In individual tumors there was some evidence of reciprocal expression of GD3 and GD2, so the combination of MAbs to GD3 and GD2 may decrease the percentage of melanoma cells that are resistant to either MAb alone.

Both GD3 and GD2, but not GM3, was expressed on lymphocytes around melanoma metastases in LNs and around melanomas in skin. GD2 was detected on a large percentage of lymphocytes around metastases in lymph nodes, but not in the skin, suggesting that the gangliosides GD2 and GD3 may be expressed on different subsets of T-lymphocytes.

These findings, together with previous studies showing that the MAbs can enhance lymphocyte responses to a variety of stimuli, provide support for the hypothesis that the clinical effects of the MAbs may reflect activation of host responses against the tumor. Further analysis of the role of gangliosides in lymphocyte function is needed.

Acknowledgments

The work of the author referred to in this chapter was supported by grants from the Hunter Valley Cancer Appeal and the National Health and Medical Research Council of Australia. I wish to thank Christine Cook for expert secretarial assistance.

References

1. Hakamori, S. (1986) Glycosphingolipids. Sci. Am. May:32–41.
2. Fishman, P.H., Brady, R.O. (1976) Biosynthesis and function of gangliosides. Science 194:906–915.
3. Markwell, M.A.K., Svennerholm, L., Paulson, J.C. (1981) Specific gangliosides function as host cell receptors for Sendai virus. Proc. Natl. Acad. Sci. USA 78:5406–5410.
4. Bergelson, L.D., Bukrinskaya, A.G., Prokazova, N.V. et al. (1982) Role of gangliosides in reception of influenza virus. Eur. J. Biochem. 128:467–474.
5. Robb. R.J. (1986) The suppressive effect of gangliosides upon IL2-dependent proliferation as a function of inhibition of IL2 receptor association. J. Immunol. 136:971.
6. Speigel, S., Fishman, P.H. (1987) Gangliosides as bimodal regulators of cell growth. Proc. Natl. Acad. Sci. USA 84:141–145.
7. Bremer, E.G., Schlessinger, J., Hakamori, S. (1986) Gangliosides mediated modulation of cell growth. Specific effects of GM3 on tyrosine phosphorylation of the epidermal growth factor receptor. J. Biol. Chem. 261:2434–2340.
8. Bremer, E.G., Hakamori, S. (1982) GM3 ganglioside induces hamster fibroblast growth inhibition in chemically defined medium: Ganglioside may regulate growth factor receptor function. Biochem. Biophys. Res. Commun. 106:711–718.
9. Goldenring, J.R., Otis, L.C., Yu, R.K., DeLorenzo, R.J. (1985) Calcium/ganglioside-dependent protein kinase activity in rat brain membrane. J. Neurochem. 44:1229–1234.
10. Spiegel, S., Panagiotopoulous, C. (1988) Mitogenesis of 3T3 fibroblasts induced by endogenous ganglioside is not mediated by cAMP, protein kinase C, or phosphoinositides turnover. Exp. Cell Res. 177(2):414–427.
11. Ravindranath, M.H., Irie, R.F. (1988) Gangliosides as antigens of human melanoma. In: Nathanson, L. ed., Cancer Treatment and Research, Vol. 4. Kluwer Academic, Norwell, MA.
12. Pukel, C.S., Lloyd, K.O., Travassos, L.R., et al. (1982) GD3, a prominent ganglioside of human melanoma. J. Exp. Med. 155:1133–1147.
13. Portoukalian, J., Zwingelstein, G., Dore, J.F. (1979) Lipid composition of human malignant melanoma tumors at various levels of malignant growth. Eur. J. Biochem. 94:19–23.
14. Cheresh, D.A., Varki, A.P., Varki, N.M., Stallcup, W.B., Levine, J., Reisfeld, R.A. (1984) A monoclonal antibody recognizes an O-acetyl sialic acid in a human melanoma-associated ganglioside. J. Biol. Chem. 259:7453–7459.

15. Furukawa, K., Chait, B.T., Lloyd, K.O. (1988) Identification of N-glycolylneuraminic acid-containing gangliosides of cat and sheep erythrocytes. J. Biol. Chem. 263:14939–14947.
16. Hellstrom, I., Brankojan, V., Hellstrom, K.E. (1985) Strong antitumor activities of IgG3 antibodies to a human melanoma associated ganglioside. Proc. Natl. Acad. Sci. USA 82: 1499–1502.
17. Cheresh, D.A., Harper, J.R., Schulz, G., Reisfeld, R.A. (1984) Localization of the gangliosides GD2 and GD3 in adhesion plaques and on the surface of human melanoma cells. Proc. Natl. Acad. Sci. USA 81:5767–5771.
18. Thurin, J., Thurin, M., Herlyn, M., et al. (1986) GD2 ganglioside biosynthesis is a distinct biochemical event in human melanoma tumor progression. FEBS Lett. 208:17–22.
19. Hirabayashi, Y., Hamaoka, A., Matsumoto, M., et al. (1985) Syngenetic monoclonal antibody against melanoma antigens with interspecies cross-reactivity recognizes GM3, a prominent ganglioside of B16 melanoma. J. Biol. Chem. 260:13328–13333.
20. Tai, T., Paulson, J.C., Cahan, L.D., Irie, R.F. (1983) Ganglioside GM2 as a human tumor antigen (OFA-1-1). Proc. Natl. Acad. Sci. USA 80:5392–5396.
21. Natoli, E.J., Livingston, P.O., Pukel, C.S., et al. (1986) A murine monoclonal antibody detecting N-acetyl- and N-glycolyl-GM2 characterization of cell surface reactivity. Cancer Res. 46:4116–4120.
22. Houghton, A.N., Mintzer, D., Cordon-Cardo, C., et al. (1985) Mouse monoclonal IgG3 antibody detecting GD3 ganlioside: A phase I trial in patients with malignant melanoma. Proc. Natl. Acad. Sci. USA 82:1242–1246.
23. Vadhan-Raj, S., Cordon-Cardo, C., Carswell, E., Mintzer, D., Dantis, L., Duteau, C., Templeton, M.A., Oettgen, H.F., Old, L.J., Houghton, A.N. (1988) Phase I trial of a mouse monoclonal antibody against GD3 ganglioside in patients with melanoma: Induction of inflammatory responses at tumor sites. J. Clin. Oncol. 6:1636–1648.
24. Cheung, N.K., Lazarus, H., Miraldi, F.D., Abramowsky, C., Kallick, S., Saaringen, U.M., Spitzer, T., Strandjord, S.E., Coccia, P.F., Berger, N.A. (1987) Ganglioside GD2 specific monoclonal antibody 3F8: A phase I study in patients with neuroblastoma and malignant melanoma. J. Clin. Oncol. 5:1430–1440.
25. Irie, R.F., Morton, D.L. (1986) Regression of cutaneous metastatic melanoma by intralesional injection with human monoclonal antibody to ganglioside GD2. Proc. Natl. Acad. Sci. USA 83:8694–8698.
26. Oldham, R.K., Foon, K.A., Morgan, C., et al. (1984) Monoclonal antibody therapy of malignant melanoma: In vivo localization in cutaneous metastases after intravenous injection. J. Clin. Oncol. 2:1235–1244.
27. Goodman, G.E., Beaumier, P., Hellstrom, I., et al. (1985) Pilot trial of murine monoclonal antibodies in patients with advanced melanoma. J. Clin. Oncol. 3:340–352.
28. Schroff, R.W., Woodhouse, C.S., Foon, K.A., Oldham, R.K., Farrell, M.M., Klein, R.A., Morgan, A.C. (1985) Intratumor localization of monoclonal antibody with melanoma treated with antibody to a 250000-Dalton melanoma-associated antigen. J. Natl. Cancer Inst. 74:299–306.
29. Hersey, P. (1989) Preclinical and phase I studies of monoclonal antibodies in melanoma. Application to boron neutron capture therapy of melanoma. Pigment Cell Res. 2:264–272.
30. Hersey, P., Schibeci, S., Townsend, P., Burns, C., Cheresh, D. (1986) Potentiation of lymphocyte responses by monoclonal antibodies to the ganglioside GD3. Cancer Res. 46:6083–6090.
31. Hersey, p., MacDonald, M., Burns, C., Cheresh, D.A. (1987) Enhancement of cytotoxic and proliferative responses of lymphocytes from melanoma patients by incubation with monoclonal antibodies against ganglioside GD3. Cancer Immunol. Immunother. 24: 144–150.
32. Welte, K., Miller, G., Chapman, P.B., et al. (1987) Stimulation of T lymphocyte proliferation by monoclonal antibodies against GD3 ganglioside. J. Immunol. 139:1763–1771.
33. Tai, T., Cahan, L.D., Tsuchida, T., Saxton, R.E., Irie, R.F., Morton, D.L. (1985) Immunogenicity of melanoma-associated gangliosides in cancer patients. Int. J. Cancer 35:607–612.

34. Cahan, L.D., Irie, R.F., Singh, R., Cassidenti, A., Paulson, J.C. (1982) Identification of a human neuroectodermal tumor antigen (OFA-1-2) as ganglioside GD2. Proc. Natl. Acad. Sci. USA 79:7629–7633.
35. Watanabe, T., Pukel, C.S., Takeyama, H., Lloyd, K.O., Shiku, H., Li, L.T.C., Travassos, L.R., Oettgen, H.F., Old, L.J. (1982) Human melanoma antigen AH is an autoantigenic ganglioside related to GD2. J. Exp. Med. 156:1884–1889.
36. Jones, P.C., Sze, L.L., Lim, P.Y., Morton, D.L., Irie, R.F. (1981) Prolonged survival for melanoma patients with elevated IgM antibody to oncofetal antigen. J. Natl. Cancer Inst. 66:249–254.
37. Portoukalian, J., Carrle, S., Dore, J.F., Rumke, P. (1989) Pilot study of immunotherapy with melanoma associated gangliosides in high-risk melanoma patients. In: 2nd Int. Conf. on Melanoma, abstract, p. 322.
38. Hersey, P., Jamal, O., Henderson, C., et al, (1988) Expression of the gangliosides GM3, GD3 and GD2 in tissue sections of normal skin, naevi, primary and metastatic melanoma. Int. J. Cancer 41:336–343.
39. Herlyn, M., Thurin, J., Balaban, G., Bennicelli, J.L., Herlyn, D., Elder, D.E., Bondi, E., Guerry, D., Nowell, P., Clark, W.H., Koprowski, H. (1985) Characteristics of cultured human melanocytes isolated from different stages of tumor progression. Cancer Res. 45: 5670–5676.
40. Rosenberg, J.M., Sander, D.J., Derango, R.E., Cheresh, D.A. (1988) Enzymatic basis for increased expression of GD3 on human melanoma cells derived from metastatic lesions. J. Clin. Lab. Anal. 2:91–100.
41. Goodman, G.E., Hellstrom, I., Hummel, D., Brodzinsky, L., Yeh, M.Y., Hellstrom, K.E. (1987) Proc. Am. Soc. Clin. Oncol. 6:A823.
42. Bajorin, D., Chapman, P., Kunicka, J., Cordon-Carlo, C., Welte, K., Mertelsmann, R., Melamed, M., Oettgen, H.F., Old, L.J., Houghton, A.N. (1987) Phase I trial of a combination of R24 mouse monoclonal antibody and recombinant interleukin-2 in patients with melanoma. Proc. Am. Soc. Clin. Oncol. 6:A827.
43. Lichtin, A., Iliopoulos, D., Guerry, D., Elder, D., Herlyn, D., Steplewski, Z. (1988) Therapy of melanoma with an antimelanoma ganglioside monoclonal antibody: A possible mechanism of a complete response (meeting abstract). In: Proc. Ann. Meet. Am. Soc. Clin. Oncol., Vol. 7, abstract, p. 958.
44. Hersey, P., Jamal, O. (1989) Expression of the gangliosides GD3 and GD2 on lymphocytes in tissue sections of melanoma. Pathology 21:51–58.
45. Cantrell, D.A., Smith, K.A. (1983) Transient expression of interleukin 2 receptors. Consequences for T cell growth. J. Exp. Med. 158:1895–1911.
46. Smith, K.A. (1984) The interleukin 2 hormone-receptor system. Lymphokine Res. 3:75.
47. Schibeci, S., Hersey, p., Cheresh, D. (1989) Potentiation of interleukin-2 production and its binding by monoclonal antibodies to the gangliosides GD3 and GD2. Cancer Immunol. Immunother. 29:109–117.
48. Hersey, P., Schibeci, S., Cheresh, D. (1989) The role of protein kinase C, intracellular calcium levels and cyclic nucleotide levels in augmentation of lymphocyte responses by monoclonal antibodies to GD3 and GD2. Cell. Immunol. 119:263–278.

9. Modulation of melanoma antigens by interferons

James L. Murray and Michael G. Rosenblum

1. Introduction

The interferons (IFNs) have been shown to have a number of pleiotropic effects in biological systems, including inhibition of cell division, modulation of differentiation, enhancement of phagocytosis, immune modulation, and altered expression of cell surface antigens [1–5]. The latter effect, modulation of antigen expression, has considerable interest for both basic scientists and clinicians as a mechanism of enhancing the amount of histocompatibility (HLA class I and class II) and tumor-associated antigens (TAA) on tumors, thereby partially circumventing tumor heterogeneity.

Since the optimal use of monoclonal antibodies (Mabs) for diagnosis and therapy is dependent to a great extent on their ability to bind to TAA, biologicals such as IFN could conceivably be used to selectively increase Mab uptake in tumors through cell surface upregulation of these antigens. Previous studies, to be expanded below, have demonstrated the enhancement of HLA class I and class II antigens on melanoma cell lines and fresh tumor specimens by in-vitro incubation with immune or gamma interferon (IFNγ), and to a lesser extent, by alpha interferon (IFNα). Other investigators have tested the effects of IFN on the regulation of melanoma-associated antigens (MAA) with significant yet less consistent results.

The purpose of this chapter will be to review the current status of IFN regulation of MAA and histocompatibility antigens. In this context, pertinent data will be presented under the following subheadings: a) in-vitro effects of IFN on expression of histocompatibility antigens, b) in-vitro effects of IFN on MAA, c) preclinical and clinical studies of IFN and Mab, and d) a summary and future directions.

2. In-vitro studies of IFN effects on melanoma antigens

2.1. In-vitro effects of IFN on HLA class I (A, B, C) and class II (DR, DP and DQ) antigens in melanoma

L. Nathanson (ed.), MELANOMA RESEARCH: GENETICS, GROWTH FACTORS, METASTASES, AND ANTIGENS.

Dolei et al. [6] were among the first to demonstrate increased expression and shedding of Ia-like (class II, HLADR) antigens, HLA-A, B, C antigens (class I), and β_2 microglobulin in a variety of normal and malignant cell lines, including two melanoma lines, M10 and M14, in the presence of human β-type interferon. A significant increase in the expression and shedding of these antigens occurred, which reached a peak after 48 hours of interferon exposure. In contrast, human α-type interferon (IFNα) caused enhanced expression and shedding of class I antigens and β_2-microglobulins but had no effect on Ia antigens. This work was confirmed and expanded by Liao et al. [7], using partially pure human leukocyte interferon (Cantell). In this instance, incubation of melanoma cell lines CaCL73-36 from a minimum of 16 hours to a maximum of 96 hours with leukocyte IFN caused a time-dependent enhancement of β_2 microglobulin. The effect of IFN on antigen expression was reversible and was independent of its effect on cell growth. A significant increase in HLA-class I antigen synthesis, as measured by the incorporation of [^{35}Se] methionine, along with enhanced sensitivity of the activity of leukocyte IFN of cells in the G_0/G_1 phase of the cell cytle, was noted by others [8]. Moreover, there was a greater correlation with enhanced HLA synthesis and IFN's antiviral effect than with its antiproliferative action.

Additional studies by Giacomini et al. [9] examined the effect of recombinant human leukocyte IFN and fibroblast IFN on MHC antigen regulation and shedding by melanoma cells. These investigators demonstrated that cell surface HLA-A, B, C antigens were enhanced by three types of recombinant leukocyte IFN species (IFNαA, αD, and αA/D), along with fibroblast IFN (IFNβ); however, shedding of the HLA-A, B, C complex occurred only with leukocyte IFN. All three species were capable of enhancing gene products in the HLA-D region, with effects on DC-1 being greater than DR. These results differ from previous studies in which naturally produced IFN were used [6,7] and may reflect differences in IFN purity and activity.

In contrast to the limited effects of leukocyte and/or fibroblast IFN on HLADR expression, there are numerous studies in the literature demonstrating significant enhancement of class II antigens by immune or gamma IFN (IFNγ) [10–19]. Ia antigens (HLADR) have been demonstrated on a proportion of cultured and uncultured melanoma cells [20], but not on melanocytes [20]. However, Ia-negative melanoma cell lines, as well as melanocytes, could be induced to express class II antigens by incubation with as little as 2 U/ml of recombinant IFNγ [10]. Interestingly, Ia antigen induction by IFNγ was not specific for melanomas, but occurred on a variety of other tumors and normal cell lines [14], as well as normal human melanocytes and nevus cells [15]. Ziai et al. [12], studied the effect of recombinant IFNγ on a melanoma clone resistant to its antiproliferative effects and found that HLA class II antigens were increased in both the resistant and the parental lines, whereas modulation of HLA class I antigens and MAA was seen only in the parental line. In essence, the data suggested that the modulation and expression of class II antigens by IFNγ occurred through mechanisms that were different from those responsible for modulation of either class I antigens or MAA. Further studies in this area revealed a dose-dependent enhancement of DR over DQ and DP antigen [16–19]. In the majority of fresh biopsy samples, long-term cell lines, and normal epidermal melanocytes the changes observed were not dependent on the cell cycle, the level of IFNγ receptors, or differentiation. Hence these findings tended to support the more frequent detection of HLA-DR over HLA-DQ and -DP antigens in melanoma lesions. These data might have relevance with respect to variations in tumor antigenicity and the effect of IFNγ on modulation of this parameter.

2.2. *In-vitro effects of IFN on MAA expression*

In contrast to numerous studies of the effects of IFN on class I and class II antigen expression, studies concerning IFN's effect on the modulation of MAA are less frequent and less convincing. Discrepancies noted in the literature, however, may relate to differences in the purity and type of IFN used, along with differences in cell lines and assay systems used. Houghton et al. [10], found no change in MAA induction by IFNγ, IFNα, or IFNβ as determined by a series of murine Mabs, M-1 through M-34, that are reactive with differentiation antigens on human melanomas and normal melanocytes. Other investigators have shown either no change or a decrease in the expression of a high Mr proteoglycan MAA found on the surface of over 90% of melanoma cell lines and fresh biopsy samples [21,22] when incubated with all three IFNs, although enhanced shedding of the antigen was observed [9]. Herlyn et al. [15] demonstrated increased shedding of both an intracytoplasmic 80-kD Mr MAA, as well as the GD_2 ganglioside MAA, when melanoma cells were incubated in vitro with IFNγ. No changes occurred in the surface expression of other MAA (proteoglycan, NGF receptor, P84Kd, p97Kd, P120Kd, p200Kd, and 80Kd).

Matsui et al. [23] used a novel approach to develop a Mab that recognized an antigen susceptible to immune modulation by IFNγ. In this case, hybridomas were constructed using spleen cells from mice immunized with IFNγ-treated melanoma cells and cloned, and supernatants were screened for their reactivity with IFNγ-treated melanoma cells. Two Mabs, CL203 and CL207, were selected that recognized a 96-kD MAA that was specifically enhanced by IFNγ in a time-dependent and concentration-dependent manner. The antigen was not modulated by either IFNα or IFNβ. The antigen was also detected in carcinoma cell lines, but at a much lower level than on melanoma cells.

Another novel MAA sensitive to regulation by IFNγ has been described by Carrel et al. [13]. The antigen, as defined by a Mab designated as Me 14-D12, was found on the surface of melanomas and other cell lines of neuroectodermal origin, such as gliomas, neuroblastomas [13], and some lymphoblastoid cell lines [24]. The antigen has been characterized as a two-chain glycoprotein of Mr 33 kD and 38 kD, respectively (gp 33–38) [24]. The gene coding for this antigen has been cloned and transfected into mouse Ltk cells [25]. Incubation of transfectants with IFNγ identified two mRNAs of 3.2 kb and 2.2 kb in primary and secondary L-cell transfectants, as well as in human melanoma cell lines expressing the antigen. The enhancement of antigen by IFNγ was retained in the transfectants and could be detected at the level of protein and in mRNA expression.

In contrast to the presence of several MAA which have been shown to be regulated by IFNγ, fewer MAA sensitive to the effects of IFNα or IFNβ have been identified to date. Liao et al. [7] were the first to demonstrate the enhancement of MAAs by leukocyte IFN, as detected by polyclonal monkey antisera. This induction of MAA was detected as early as 16 hours and was maximal at 96 hours after IFN exposure. Other investigators have shown that recombinant leukocyte and fibroblast IFN were also capable of increasing the surface expression and shedding of several intracytoplasmic antigens of 115 kD and 100 kD, respectively [9].

Murray et al. [22] studied the in-vitro effects of recombinant IFNα and IFNγ on the modulation of the transferrin-like glycoprotein P97, as well as the high molecular weight (240 kD) proteoglycan. P97, a 97 kD Mr surface antigen, is found on over 80% of melanoma cell lines and fresh human melanomas, and has minimal cross-reactivity with endothelial cells and fetal tissues [26]. The 240 kD Mr antigen is found on over 90% of melanoma cell lines and fresh biopsy specimens [21]. Melanoma cell line HS294t [27] was incubated with either 50, 500, or 1000 U/ml IFNα, IFNγ, or a combination of the two for 4, 24, 48, and 72 hours at 37°C in flat-bottomed microtiter plates (30–50,000 cells/well). Following incubation, media was removed and Mabs 96.5 or ZME018, reactive with P97 or proteoglycan antigen, respecitvely, were added at an optimal concentration of 1 μg/ml. After 1 hour incubation at 37°C, plates were again washed and a saturating amount of ^{125}I-labeled goat anti-mouse IgG (specific activity 10 μCi/μg was added. Following three additional washes, cells were lysed with detergent, total counts were absorbed using cotton swabs, and the total counts per minute per 10^5 cells was determined by gamma counting. As shown in Table 1, preincubation of cells with either 500 U/ml of IFNα or IFNγ for 48 hours significantly enhanced binding of Mab 96.5 over cells preincubated in media alone. Higher or lower concentrations of IFN for shorter or longer time periods did not have a significantly greater effect. In contrast, surface expression of the 240 kD antigen was not modulated by either IFN, similar to what has been reported previously [9]. IFN also enhanced HLADR expression slightly and did not affect binding of an irrelevant Mab, OKT_3 (Table 1). No effects of IFNα or IFNγ were observed using a breast carcinoma cell line, MCF-7.

The effects of a combination of each IFN on P97 antigen expression was also studied. Addition of 250 U/ml IFNα to 250 U/ml IFNγ did not significantly enhance antigen expression to a significantly greater extent than 500 U/ml of each respective IFN alone, indicating that the two IFNs were not synergistic and in some cases were less than additive. As demonstrated pre-

Table 1. Specificity of MoAb binding and regulation by IFN

Cell line	IFN (500 U/ml)	Antibody added				
		^{125}I-GAMIgG[a]	96.5	ZME018	OKIa[b]	OKT3[c]
HS294t	0	2518 ± 547	7408 ± 118	7149 ± 118	32914 ± 1584	4304 ± 609
	rIFNα-A	–	10696 ± 87[e]	9297 ± 1063	33409 ± 1895	4611 ± 180
	$rIFN_y$	–	12596 ± 717[e]	8801 ± 1006	39284 ± 813[f]	3499 ± 332
MCF-7[d]	0	1097 ± 200	1315 ± 62	2024 ± 272	NT	NT
(control)	rIFNα-A	–	1051 ± 64	2310 ± 5	–	–
	$rIFN_y$	–	1628 ± 161	1903 ± 243	–	–

Values represent mean ± SEM cmp MoAb bound/10^5 cells from three experiments following 48 hours incubation of tumor cells with IFN. NT = not tested.

[a] Represents tumor cells incubated with ^{125}I-labeled goat anti-mouse IgG alone.

[b] OKIa = MoAb recognizing HLADR.

[c] OKT3 = MoAb recognizing pan-T cell antigen.

[d] MCF-7 = breast carcinoma cell line.

[e] Significant increase over baseline. $p < 0.001$.

[f] Significant at $p < 0.025$ vs. baseline.

From Murray et al. (1988) J. Biol. Response Modifiers, 7:152–161, with publisher's permission.

viously [28], synergistic inhibition of proliferation by a combination of each IFN occurred, indicating that IFN's effects on antigen modulation were disassociated from its effects on cell growth.

In summary, the majority of in-vitro studies have demonstrated variable effects of IFNs on melanoma surface antigen modulation depending on several parameters including the antigen, the concentration of IFN, the length of incubation, the assay procedure(s), and melanoma cell lines used. Hence, direct comparisons of findings from different investigators are difficult and are fraught with errors in interpretation.

3. Preclinical and clinical studies of Mabs and IFN

Several studies have demonstrated an enhancement of tumor targeting of Mabs in vivo in nude mice given IFNα or IFNγ [29,30]. The Mabs used were those recognizing breast cancer (B6) or HLADR antigen (Tal-1B5); IFNα was injected into mice receiving B6 Mab and IFNγ into mice receiving TAL-1B5. In both studies, improved tumor localization was antigen specific, since isotype-matched irrelevant Mabs did not accumulate within tumors of either control or recombinant IFN-treated mice.

There is little data regarding the effect of IFN in vivo on Mab targeting in mice bearing melanoma xenografts. Murray et al., as a follow-up to data showing a 40–70% enhancement of P97 on melanoma cells treated with recombinant IFNα in vitro [22], performed a study of 96.5 localization in athymic mice bearing established subcutaneous tumors comprised of HS294t human melanoma cells [31]. Tumor-bearing mice were given single daily intramuscular injections of either normal saline or IFNα (subspecies A) at concentrations of 5×10^3, 30×10^3, or 250×10^3 U for a total of 10 days. On day 7, mice received 5 μg of either ^{111}In-labeled Mab 96.5 or the irrelevant subclass-matched ^{111}In-labeled Mabs T101 and ZCE025 (an anti-T-cell Mab and anti-CEA Mab, respectively). Animals were sacrificed 72 hours later, and the percent injected dose per gram (%1D/g) in tumors and normal organs was determined. Mabs T101 and ZCE025 did not localize specifically to melanoma tissues, as demonstrated by tissue to blood ratios of 0.5 compared to a tissue to blood ratio of 5 for the specific antibody 96.5. As shown in Table 2, there was a significant ($p < .001$) increase of 96.5 in tumors of IFNα-treated mice compared to saline-treated controls. Targeting of control Mabs was not significantly enhanced by IFNα. An interesting finding of this study was that IFNα treatment also increased the %ID/g 96.5 in normal tissues, chiefly blood, heart, lung, and kidney. Analysis of homogenized tissue specimens for antigen revealed the presence of P97 in these tissues, especially in IFN-treated mice. These data were compatible with either IFNα causing enhanced tumor shedding of antigen with localization in tissues, or the enhanced expression of an antigen that cross-reacts with 96.5 in normal tissues. It is known that P97 is similar in structure to transferrin [32] and is

Table 2. Tumor uptake of ^{111}In-96.5 vs. control MABs in control vs rIFNαA treated mice

^{111}In-MAB	NS (control)	rIFNαA (U/day × 10 days)		
		5000	30,000	250,000
96.5	12.0 ± 1.8[a]	30.8 ± 5.5[b]	36.0 ± 4.7[b]	29.4 ± 10.5
T101 (control)	4.3 ± 0.9	N.D.[c]	4.7 ± 1.2	3.8 ± 0.62
ZCE025	6.9 ± 0.9	N.D.[c]	15.0 ± 4	N.D.[c]

[a] Data represent mean ± SEM % inj. dose/g of MAB. In from 5–12 mice/GP.
[b] $p < .001$ vs. NS control mice.
[c] N.D. = not done.

found to a limited extent on endothelial cells [33]. Additional studies are needed to determine the relevance of these findings.

Matsui et al. [34] performed an interesting study in which an immunoconjugate of CL207 (recognizing the IFNγ-regulated 96 kD MAA) and daunomycin displayed a selective in-vitro cytotoxic effect against melanoma cells expressing the antigen. IFNγ caused a synergistic enhancement of selective immunoconjugate cytotoxicity. Furhermore, in mice bearing BM-314 colon carcinoma cells (CL202 reacts with both melanomas and carcinomas), tumor growth was significantly inhibited in animals receiving IFNγ plus conjugate versus animals treated with conjugate alone, IFNγ alone, CL207 alone, or a mixture of daunomycin and CL207. These studies, coupled with the data presented above, suggest a possible role for the use of combinations of IFN and Mabs in the diagnosis and therapy of cancer in humans.

3.1. A pilot clinical trial of a combination of leukocyte IFN and Mab 96.5 in humans

To determine whether IFN could influence the pharmacokinetics as well as the biodistribution of anti melanoma Mab in humans, we performed a pilot clinical trial in which melanoma patients (n = 5) were selected to receive partially purified leukocyte IFN (HUIFNα-Cantell), followed by an infusion of ^{111}In-labeled murine antimelanoma antibody, 96.5 [35]. The antibody chosen was based on our earlier preclinial results in vitro, which demonstrated an enhancement of surface antigen P97 by both recombinant IFNα and IFNγ [22]. Results in the above patients were compared to five patients who received ^{111}In-96.5 alone as part of a larger phase III radioimaging study (controls). Although patients were not randomized, the distribution of patient characteristics, including mean age, sex, previous treatment, and histories, was similar in both groups. Patients were also matched with respect to the mean diameter of soft tissue lesions (i.e., lymph nodes, skin), as measured in centimeters. Controls had a greater number of documented lymph node and visceral metastases (n = 23) than HuIFNα-treated patients (n = 6).

Prior to study, all patients gave written informed consent, as required by the Surveillance Committee at University of Texas M.D. Anderson Cancer Center. Computerized axial tomography scans of brian, abdomen, and pelvis, along with other routine radiographs, were performed to completely document metastatic disease. Five patients were begun on HuIFNα, 3×10^6 U daily by intramuscular injection. HuIFNα treatment was continued as long as disease stabilization or a response to therapy was evident.

Twenty-four hours after receiving the first injection of HuIFNα, patients were given 1 mg of ^{111}In-labeled 96.5, along with 19 mg of unlabeled 96.5 in 100 ml of normal saline as a 1-hour infusion. The dose selected had been demonstrated to give optimal imaging in a previous phase I trial [36]. Seventy-two hours following Mab infusion (i.e., day 4 of HuIFNα treatment), gamma scans were performed using a GE model 400 gamma camera (Milwaukee, WI), and images were stored in an on-line computer (Digital-Gamma II, DEC, Maynard, MA). Patients not receiving HuIFNα were given Mab alone and imaged in the same fashion. Scans were initially interpreted by a single nuclear medicine physician without full knowledge of disease sites.

To determine the relative uptakes of ^{111}In-labeled 96.5 in tumor with respect to background, regions of interest (ROIs) were drawn on the digital images taken at 72 hours postinjection over the bones (lumbar spine), kidneys, spleen, and the largest soft tissue lesion. Lesions were restrospectively matched for size and site between HuIFNα-treated patients and controls. These were compared to ROIs over the liver and heart using average counts per pixel. When image collection was different from the standard 5 minutes, equalization was achieved first. Counts were also corrected to a standard grid format of 64×64. If any visceral organ contained tumor, these were avoided in drawing ROIs.

The plasma half-life of ^{111}In-labeled 96.5 was determined by analyzing counts per minute from heparinized 5 ml blood samples collected during ^{111}In Mab infusion, at the end of infusion (time 0), and at 1, 5, 10, 30, 60, 70, 120, 180, 1320, and 2760 minutes after infusion. An aliquot (0.5 ml) of the ^{111}In-labeled Mab solution was also obtained to serve as a standard and isotope decay control. Blood samples were centrifuged and duplicate 100-μl aliquots of plasma were added to 13×100 mm disposable glass test tubes. Radioactivity was assessed using a Packard scintillation gamma counter (model 5360).

The results of this study were as follows. First, although the number of patients in this study was small, there was a significant difference in the number and percentage of metastases imaged in the HuIFNα group compared to the controls (HuIFNα: 21 of 27 (78%); controls: 23 of 42 (55%), P = .05, chi square). The increase in imaging was due to a significantly greater detection of lung lesions; detection of skin and soft tissue lesions, visceral lesions, and lymph nodes was not significantly different between the two groups (68% vs. 67% in the HuIFNα group vs. controls, respectively). ROI scans for representative patients who received 96.5 antibody without prior IFN treatment (Figure 1A) or after IFN are shown (Figure 1B). With IFN treatment, there was a greater distribution of the label to tumor and to peripheral tissues.

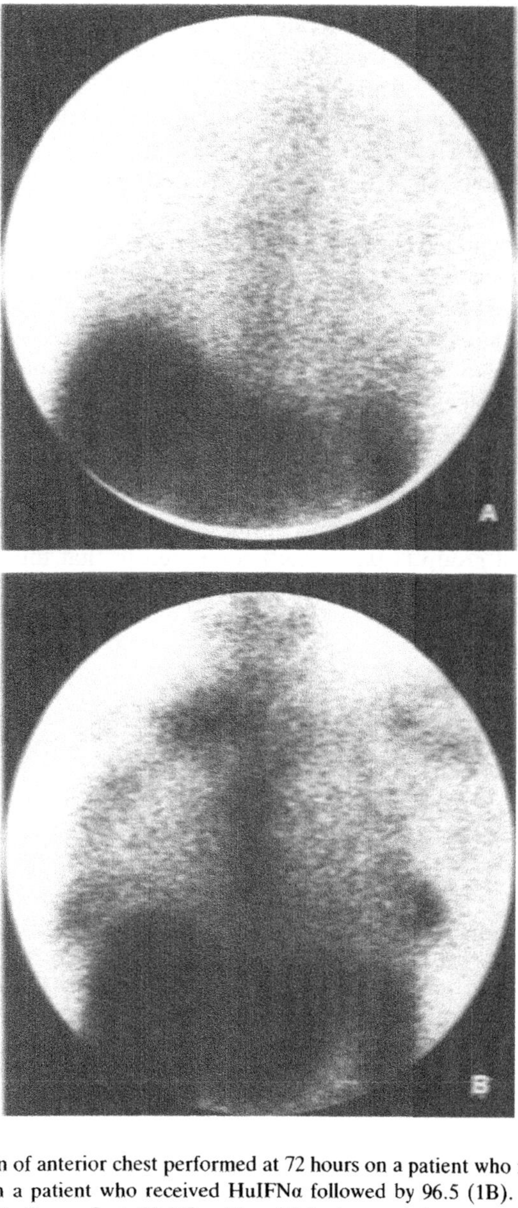

Figure 1. ROI scan of anterior chest performed at 72 hours on a patient who received Mab 96.5 alone (1A) and on a patient who received HuIFNα followed by 96.5 (1B). From Rosenblum (1988) et al. J. Natl. Cancer Inst. 80:160, with publisher's permission.

Figure 2 shows the mean plasma concentration of [^{111}In] from the five patients who received antibody 96.5 alone compared to the group receiving 96.5 and HuIFNα. With the same dose of both antibody and [^{111}In] label, the HuIFNα-treated group displayed a 50% decrease in the concentration of radiolabel in plasma compared to controls early after the end of infusion (time 0). However, the rate of clearance of radiolabel from plasma appeared to be slower for the HuIFNα-treated group than for controls. As indicated in Figure 1, the HuIFNα-treated group demonstrated a substantial increase in $t_{1/2}$ (from 19.8 ± 3.2 hours to 39.7 ± 3.3 hours) compared to controls. In addition, the decrease in concentration of the radiolabel in the blood pool observed in Figure 1 was reflected in a concomitant increase in the apparent volume of distribution of the HuIFNα-treated group compared to that of controls.

In light of the above findings, a comparison was made between the relative amount of radioactivity in tumor sites versus blood pool and other organ sites, including liver, spleen, kidneys, and bone. ROIs were selected on 72-hour scans and the counts per minute per pixel was determined for a representative soft-tissue lesion and for each of the above organs. Soft-tissue lesions of similar size and location on the body surface were selected in order to minimize differences due to depth and gamma camera scanning angle. A ratio of counts per minute per pixel in tumor versus heart (blood pool), as well as other organs versus heart, was calculated for each patient. As shown in Figure 3, there was a significant increase in the mean ± SEM tumor/blood ratio in the IFN-treated group (1.98 ± 0.68) compared to that found in the control

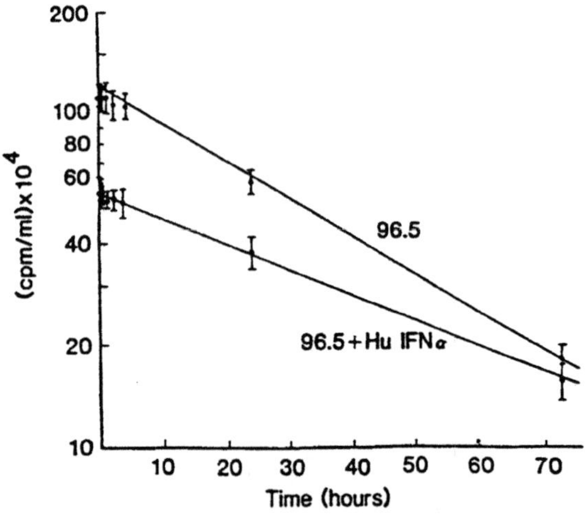

Figure 2. $T_{1/2}$ of 96.5 in controls and HuIFNα-treated patients. The calculated line was monophasic in both instances. Solic lines represent the best-fit, least squares regression line through these points. Values shown are means for five patients per group ± SEM. From Rosenblum et al. (1988) J. Natl. Cancer Inst. 80:160, with publisher's permission.

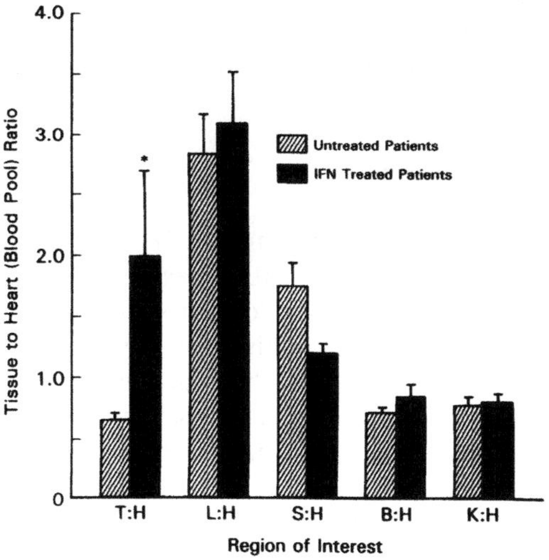

Figure 3. Mean ± SEM ratios of antibody in tumor (T), liver (L), spleen (S), bone (B), and kidney (K) relative to heart (H) or blood pool. * = significant at $p < .05$.

group (0.63 ± 0.06). However, in liver, spleen, bone, and kidney, there were no significant differences in antibody content between controls and the IFN-treated group. Tumors in the HuIFNα group had a higher average radioactivity expressed as counts per pixel (438.4 ± 101.8) than tumor in the control group (276.6 ± 48: p = .06). Relative counts per pixel in blood pool and in other organs were comparable between groups. When the relative counts per minute were expressed as a ratio to counts per minute in liver, there was a statistically significant increase in the amount of radiolabel distributed to the tumor in the IFN-treated group (data not shown).

Although this represents the first clinical study to demonstrate significant alterations in anti-melanoma Mab pharmacokinetics and biodistribution by alpha interferon species, the data should be interpreted with caution. First, because biopsies could not be obtained in the patients and an irrelevant subclass-matched Mab was not given, one cannot conclude that the enhanced localization of ^{111}-labeled 96.5 was specific or was due to enhanced antigen expression on the tumor. However, it is of interest that the prolonged clearance of Mab in the IFN group, coupled with an increase in the volume of distribution (Figures 1 and 2), parallels our findings in nude mice with respect to increased 96.5 in tissues [31]. In an earlier study, circulating P97 was measured in 1 of 20 patients receiving ^{111}In-labeled 96.5 alone [37], hence it is theoretically possible that enhanced antigen shedding and/or upregulation in normal tissues by IFN is occurring. The existence of a saturable P97 antigen pool in normal human tissues has been demonstrated by the ability of 'cold' or unlabeled 6.5 given concomitantly or prior to 1 mg ^{111}In-labeled Mab to block liver uptake of labeled 96.5 and to enhance tumor uptake of the same

[38]. Despite evidence favoring antigen-mediated uptake, further trials are needed using a control nonspecific Mab as well as biopsies, both pre- and post-IFN treatment, to confirm these results.

4. Summary and future directions

The above studies have shown that human IFN, both alpha and gamma species, were capable of enhancing antigen expression and/or shedding, as detected by a variety of Mabs specific for histocompatibility and melanoma-associated antigens. The degree of modulation was variable and appeared to be dependent on the antigen studied, the concentration of IFN, the time of incubation, the cell lines used, and the assay systems employed. It was nevertheless encouraging to see that in-vitro results could be preliminarily confirmed in-vivo in nude mice, as well as in humans. However, we should continue to use caution in interpreting the results of in-vivo studies suggesting an enhancement of tumor targeting secondary to antigen upregulation alone, since Mab uptake in tumors is due to a host of variables, including tumor blood flow, permeability, and antibody charge [39,40].

Although the in-vitro results are interesting, future studies should concentrate on whether modulation of a particular antigen has any functional of biological significance. In terms of regulation of class I and class II histocompatibility antigens, the IFNs may serve as important modulators of tumor immunogenicity with respect to antigen-specific cellular and tumoral immunity in vivo. In addition, the three types of IFN have been shown to significantly enhance the expression of an intracellular adhesion molecule on metastatic and nonmetastatic melanoma cell lines, the former to a greater extent that the latter [41]. These findings may have particular relevance with respect to IFN influencing the degree of metastatic potential of tumors and inhibition by Mabs against these antigens.

Additional in-vitro and in-vivo studies should examine the potential for various combinations of cytokines and/or differentiating agents in synergistically enhancing relevant antigens. With the advent of clinical trials using combinations of Mabs and cytokines (i.e., IL-2, IFN), it is important to understand the effects of these molecules at the tumor cell, as well as the cytotoxic effector cell level. For example, downregulation of a particular antigen by IFN might influence an effector cell's ability to mediate antibody-dependent cell-mediated cytotoxicity due to a lack of sufficient antibody at the tumor site.

Additional studies examining the role of IFN with respect to antigen regulation at the molecular level need to be pursued. The inducement of relevant antigens on antigen-negative variants via gene amplification remains an exciting area of research [25] and could have significant therapeutic and immunologic consequences.

Lastly, with respect to the clinical relevance to these findings, more studies should be designed to address whether antigen modulation can have a sufficient influence on Mab distribution in patients. Presurgical studies in which relevant and irrelevant Mabs are given and biopsies are taken to determine the amount of respective Mab bound to tumors in patients treated with interferon versus those not receiving IFN need to be performed to prove this hypothesis. These trials are difficult to design and contain ethical considerations, particularly in the instance in which the same patient would serve as his or her own control (i.e., have two biopsies performed, one pre- and one post-IFN and Mab treatment). For antibodies that mediate effector functions, as well as bind to antigens that are modulated by IFN, the overall effect of their combination needs to be considered. Despite these complexities, studies performed to data that suggest a role for the IFNs in antigen modulation are encouraging and might serve as one of several methods of enhancing Mab delivery to the tumor site, as well as serve as a focal point for understanding the complex genetic mechanisms underlying tumor antigen regulation in humans.

Acknowledgments

This work was supported in part by PHS grant CA-43544 from the National Cancer Institute and Hybritech, Incorporated.

References

1. Matarese, G.P., Rossi, G.B. (1978) Effect of interferon on growth and division cycle of Friend erythroleukemic cells in vitro. J. Cell Biol. 75:344–355.
2. Dolei, A., Colletta, G., Capobranchi, M.R., et al. (1980) Interferon effects of Friend leukemia cells. I-Expression of viral and erythoid markets in undetected and dimethylsulfoxide treated cells. J. Gen. Virol. 46:227–236.
3. Huang, E., Donahue, R.M., Gordon, F.B., et al. (1971) Enhancement of phagocytosis by interferon-containing preparation. Infect. Immun. 4:581–588.
4. Trinchieri, G., Santoli, D. (1978) Enhancement of human natural killer cell activity by interferon. J. Immunol. 120:1845–1850.
5. Gresser, I. (1977) On the varied biologic effects of interferon. Cell Immunol. 34:406–411.
6. Dolei, A., Ameglio, F., Capobianchi, M.R., et al. (1981) Human β-type interferon enhances the expression and shedding of Ia-like antigens, comparison to HLA-A, B, C and β_s-microglobulin. Antiviral Res. 1:367–381.
7. Liao, S-K., Kwong, P.C., Khosravi,M. (19) Enhanced expression of melanoma-associated antigens and β_2-microglobulin on cultured human melanoma cells by interferon. J. Natl. Cancer Inst. 68(1):19–25.
8. Basham, T.Y., Bourgeade, M.F., Creasey, A.A. (1982) Interferon increases HLA synthesis in melanoma cells: Interferon-resistant and -sensitive cell lines. Proc. Natl. Acad. Sci. USA 79(5):3265–3269.
9. Giacomini, P., Aguzzi, A., Pestka, S., et al. (1984) Modulation by recombinant DNA leukocyte (α) and fibroblast (β) interferons of the expression and shedding of HLA- and tumor-associated antigens by human melanoma cells. J. Immunol. 133(3):1649–1655.

10. Houghton, A.N., Thomson, T.M., Gross, D., et al. (1984) Surface antigens of melanoma and melanocytes: Specificity of induction of Ia antigens by human γ-interferon. J. Exp. Med. 160(7):255–269.
11. Giacomini, P., Imberti, L., Aguzzi, A., et al. (1985) Immunochemical analysis of the modulation of human melanoma-associated antigens by DNA recombinant immune interferon. J. Immunol. 135(4):2887–2894.
12. Ziai, M.R., Imberti, L., Tongson, A., et al. (1985) Differential modulation by recombinant immune interferon of the expression and shedding of HLA antigens and melanoma associated antigens by a melanoma cell line resistant to the antiproliferative activity of immune interferon. Cancer Res. 45(11):5877–5882.
13. Carrel, S., Schmidt-Kessen, A., Giuffre, L. (1985) Recombinant interferon-γ can induce the expression of HLA-DR and -DC on DR-negative melanoma cells and enhance the expression of HLA-ABC and tumor-associated antigens. Eur. J. Immunol. 15:118–123.
14. Shaw, A.R.E., Chan, J.K.W., Reid, S., et al. (1985) HLA-DR synthesis induction and expression in HLA-DR-negative carcinoma cell lines of diverse origins by interferon-γ but not by interferon-β. J. Natl. Cancer Inst. 74(6):1261–1267.
15. Herlyn, M., Guerry, D., Koprowski, H. (1985) Recombinant γ- interferon induces changes in expression and shedding of antigens associated with normal human melanocytes, nevus cells, and primary and metastatic melanoma cells. J. Immunol. 134(6):4226–4230.
16. Tarmelli, D., Fossati, G., Mazzocchi, A., et al. (1986) Classes I and II HLA and melanoma-associated antigen expression and modulation on melanoma cells isolated from primary and metastatic lesions. Cancer Res. 46(1):433–439.
17. Anichini, A., Mortarini, R., Fossati, G., et al. (1986) Phenotypic profile of clones from early cultures of human metastatic melanomas and its modulation by recombinant interferonγ. Int. J. Cancer 38:505–511.
18. Tsujisaki, M., Igarashi, M., Sakaguchi, K., et al. (1987) immunochemical and functional analysis of HLA class II antigens induced by recombinant immune interferon on normal epidermal melanocytes. J. Immunol. 238(4)1310–1316.
19. Anichini, A., Castelli, C., Sozzi, G., et al. (1988) Differential susceptibility to recombinant interferon-γ-induced HLA-DQ antigen modulation among clones from a human metastatic melanoma. J. Immunol. 140(1):183–191.
20. Houghton, A.N., Eisinger, M., Albino,A.P., et al. (1982) Surface antigens of melanocytes and melanomas. Markers of melanocyte differentiation and melanoma subsets. J. Exp. Med. 156:1735–1766.
21. Ng, A.K., Giacomini, P., Kantor, R., et al. (1982) Molecular heterogeneity and shedding of a high molecular weight melanoma-associated antigen identified with monoclonal antibodies. Clin. Chem. 28(12):2347–2350.
22. Murray, J.L., Stuckey, S.E., Pillow, J.K., et al. (1988) Differential in vitro effects of recombinant α-interferon and recombinant γ-interferon alone or in combination on the expression of melanoma-associated surface antigens. J. Biol. Response Mod. 7:152–161.
23. Matsui, M., Temponi, M., Ferrone,S. (1987) Characterization of a monoclonal antibody-defined human melanoma-associated antigen susceptible to induction by immune interferon. J. Immunol. 139:(9)2088–2095.
24. Guiggre, L., Isler, P., Schreyer, M., et al. (1988) A novel interferon-γ regulated human melanoma-associated antigen, gp33–38, defined by monoclonal antibody Me14-D12.I. Identification and immunochemical characterization. J. Immunol. 141:2072–2078.
25. Audette, M., Carrel, S., Hayoz, D., et al. (1989) A novel interferon-γ regulated human melanoma-associated antigen, gp33–38, defined by monoclonal antibody Me14-D12, II. Molecular cloning of a genomic probe. Molecular Immunol. 26(6):515–522.
26. Brown, J.P., Nishiyama, K., Hellstrom, I., et al. (1981) Structural characterization of human melanoma-associated antigen P97 with monoclonal antibodies. J. Immunol. 127:539–546.
27. Creasy, A.A., Smith, H.S., Hacket, A.J., et al. (1979) Biological properties of human melanoma cells in culture. In vitro 15:342–350.
28. Schiller, J.H., Groveman, D.S., Schmid, S.M., et al. (1986) Synergistic antiproliferative

effects of human recombinant α54- or βser-interferon with γ-interferon on human cell lines of various histogenesis. Cancer Res. 46(2):483–488.

29. Greiner, J.W., Guadagni, F., Noguchi, P., et al. (1987) Recombinant interferon enhances monoclonal antibody-targeting of carcinoma lesions in vivo. Science 235(2):895–898.
30. Rowlinson, G., Balkwill, F., Snook, D., et al. (1987) Enhancement by γ-interferon of *in vivo* tumor radiolocalization by a monoclonal antibody against HLA-DR antigen. Cancer Res. 46:6413–6417.
31. Murray, J.L., Zukiwski, A.A., Rosenblum, M.G. (1989) Enhanced tumor targeting of ^{111}In-labeled murine anti-melanoma monoclonal antibody (Mab) 96.5 in nude mice receiving recombinant alpha interferon, subspecies A(rIFNαA). Proc. Am. Assoc. Cancer Res. 30.
32. Brown,J.P., Harwick, R.M., Hellstrom, I., et al. (1982) Human melanoma-associated antigen P97 is structurally and functionally related to transferrin. Nature (London) 296: 171–173.
33. Brown, J.P., Woodbury,R.G., Hunt, C.E., et al. (1981) Identification of a cell surface protein, P97, in human melanoma and certain other neoplasms. Proc. Natl. Acad. Sci. 78.
34. Matsui, M., Nakanishi, T., Noguchi, T., et al. (1988) Synergistic *in vitro* and *in vivo* antitumor effect of daunomycin-anti-96kDa melanoma-associated antigen monoclonal antibdoy CL207 conjugate and recombinant IFNγ. J. Immunol. 141(8):1410–1417.
35. Rosenblum, M.G., Lamki, L.M., Murray, J.L., et al. (1988) Interferon-induced changes in pharmacokinetics and tumor uptake of ^{111}In-labeled antimelanoma antibody 96.5 in melanoma patients. J. Natl. Cancer Inst. 80(4):160–165.
36. Murray, J.L., Rosenblum, M.G., Sobol, R.E., et al. (1985) Radioimmunoimaging in malignant melanoma with ^{111}In-labeled monoclonal antibody 96.5. Cancer Res. 45:3476–2381.
37. Murray, J.L., Hersh, E.M., Rosenblum, M., et al. (1985) Radioimmunoimaging in malignant melanoma using ^{111}indium-labeled anti-P-97 monoclonal antibody. In: Chatterjee S., ed., Monoclonal Antibodies, Diagnostic and Therapeutic Use in Tumor and Transplantation. PSG Publishing, Littleton, MA, pp. 143–153.
38. Murray, J.L., Lamki, L.M., Shanken, L.J., et al. (1988) Immunospecific saturable clearance mechanisms for ^{111}indium-labeled anti-melanoma monoclonal antibody 96.5 in humans. Cancer Res. 48(8):4417–4422.
39. Sands, H., Jones, P.L., Shah, S.A., et al. (1988) Correlation of vascular permeability and blood flow with monoclonal antibody uptake by human Clouser and renal cell xenografts. Cancer Res. 48(1):188–193.
40. Haskell, C.M., Bucheggar, F., Schreyer, F., et al. (1983) Monoclonal antibodies to carcinoembryonic antigen: Ionic strength as a factor in the selection of antibodies for immunoscintigraphy. Cancer Res. 43:3857–3864.
41. Maio, M., Gulwani, B., Langer, J.A., et al. (1989) Modulation for interferons of HLA antigen, high-molecular-weight melanoma-associated antigen, and intercellular adhesion molecule 1 expression by cultured melanoma cells with different metastatic potential. Cancer Res. 49(6):2980–2987.

Index

GPSR Compliance

The European Union's (EU) General Product Safety Regulation (GPSR) is a set of rules that requires consumer products to be safe and our obligations to ensure this.

If you have any concerns about our products, you can contact us on ProductSafety@springernature.com

In case Publisher is established outside the EU, the EU authorized representative is:

Springer Nature Customer Service Center GmbH
Europaplatz 3
69115 Heidelberg, Germany

Batch number: 10755292

Printed by Printforce, the Netherlands